# Chinese Medicated Liquor Therapy

# 中 国 酒 疗

**Chief-editor： Song Nong**
**Translator： Li Guohua**

**Beijing Science & Technology Press**
北京科学技术出版社

**First Edition** 1996
ISBN 7-5304-1845-9/R · 356

Chinese Medicated Liquor Therapy
Chief-editor   Song Nong
Translator   Li Guohua
Published by
Beijing Science & Technology Press
16 Xizhimen Nandajie, Beijing 100035, China

Distributed by
China International Book Trading Corporation
35 Chegongzhuang Xilu, Beijing 100044, China
P.O. Box 399, Beijing, China

*Printed in the People's Republic of China*

# Preface

　　Chinese Medicated Liquor Therapy is specially written for those foreign friends who sant to study traditional Chinese Medicine. In this book, hundreds of prescriptions have been discussed. Th ingredients, process, directions and indications of each prescription have been concisely described. Medicated liquor therpy here refers to not only the method of by using traditional medicated liquor, but also the treatment concerning with alcoholic drinkds under the guidance of traditional Chinese medicine. The names of most diseases are those of the symptoms and syndromes according to the habitudes of traditional Chinese medicine.

The editor

# CONTENTS

## Chapter One   Internal Diseases

| | | |
|---|---|---|
| Section 1 | Fever | (5) |
| Section 2 | Headache | (6) |
| Section 3 | Common Cold and Influenza | (10) |
| Section 4 | Cough | (13) |
| Section 5 | Pulmonary Abscess | (20) |
| Section 6 | Asthma | (21) |
| Section 7 | Dyspepsia | (24) |
| Section 8 | Anorexia | (29) |
| Section 9 | Vomiting | (30) |
| Section 10 | Hiccup | (34) |
| Section 11 | Epigastric Pain | (35) |
| Section 12 | Abdominal Pain | (40) |
| Section 13 | Pain in the Chest and Hypochondria | (45) |
| Section 14 | Diarrhea | (49) |
| Section 15 | Jaundice | (53) |
| Section 16 | Spontaneous Perspiration and Night Sweat | (54) |
| Section 17 | Constipation | (56) |
| Section 18 | Angina Pectoris | (60) |
| Section 19 | Hypertension | (62) |
| Section 20 | Hyperlipemia | (64) |
| Section 21 | Hypotension | (64) |
| Section 22 | Anemia | (66) |
| Section 23 | Edema | (67) |
| Section 24 | Paruria | (69) |
| Section 25 | Nephritis | (73) |
| Section 26 | Renal Tuberculosis | (74) |
| Section 27 | Impotency | (75) |
| Section 28 | Premature Ejaculation | (82) |
| Section 29 | Emission | (83) |

| | | |
|---|---|---|
| Section 30 | Simple Goiter | (91) |
| Section 31 | Diabetes Mellitus | (92) |
| Section 32 | Hemiplegia | (94) |
| Section 33 | Epilepsy | (98) |
| Section 34 | Melancholy | (100) |
| Section 35 | Amnesia | (103) |
| Section 36 | Insomnia | (105) |
| Section 37 | Parotitis | (109) |
| Section 38 | Malaria | (111) |
| Section 39 | Dysentery | (113) |

## Chapter Two   Surgical Diseases

| | | |
|---|---|---|
| Section 1 | Furuncle, Carbuncle and Cellulitis | (117) |
| Section 2 | Lymphadenitis | (120) |
| Section 3 | Lymphoid Tuberculosis | (121) |
| Section 4 | Osseous Tuberculosis | (122) |
| Section 5 | Mastitis | (123) |
| Section 6 | Angiitis | (125) |
| Section 7 | Hernia | (125) |
| Section 8 | Hemorrhoids | (126) |
| Section 9 | Prolapse of Rectum | (127) |
| Section 10 | Bi Syndrome | (128) |
| Section 11 | Sciatica | (148) |
| Section 12 | Fracture | (150) |
| Section 13 | Scapulohumeral Periarthritis | (152) |
| Section 14 | Traumatic Injury | (153) |

## Chapter Three
## Gynecologic and Obstetric Diseases

| | | |
|---|---|---|
| Section 1 | Irregular Menstruation | (164) |
| Section 2 | Dysmenorrhea | (171) |
| Section 3 | Amenorrhea | (173) |
| Section 4 | Metrorrhagia | (175) |
| Section 5 | Abnormal Leukorrhea | (177) |

| Section 6 | Infertility | (180) |
| Section 7 | Threatened Abortion | (182) |
| Section 8 | Retention of Placenta | (184) |
| Section 9 | Postpartum Abdominal Pain | (185) |
| Section 10 | Postpartum Hemorrhage | (188) |
| Section 11 | Lochiorhea | (191) |
| Section 12 | Galactostasis | (192) |
| Section 13 | Hypogalactia | (194) |
| Section 14 | Prolapse of Uterus | (197) |
| Section 15 | Other Proved Prescriptions for Postpartum Syndromes | (199) |

## Chapter Four  Pediatric Diseases

| Section 1 | Hernia | (204) |
| Section 2 | Erysipelas | (205) |
| Section 3 | Eczema | (205) |
| Section 4 | Enuresis | (206) |
| Section 5 | Vomiting | (206) |
| Section 6 | Common Cold | (207) |
| Section 7 | Pertussis | (208) |
| Section 8 | Varicella | (208) |

## Chapter Five
## Diseases of Eyes, Ears, Nose and Throat

| Section 1 | Conjunctivitis | (209) |
| Section 2 | Eye Injury | (209) |
| Section 3 | Nyctalopia | (210) |
| Section 4 | Piminution of Vision | (211) |
| Section 5 | Pharyngitis | (212) |
| Section 6 | Acute Tonsillitis | (212) |
| Section 7 | Aphonia | (213) |
| Section 8 | Paranasal Sinusitis | (214) |
| Section 9 | Epistaxis | (214) |
| Section 10 | Tympanitis | (215) |
| Section 11 | Toothache | (216) |

## Chapter Six  Dermatoses

| | | |
|---|---|---|
| Section 1 | Urticaria | (218) |
| Section 2 | Psoriasis | (219) |
| Section 3 | Frostbite | (220) |
| Section 4 | Vitiligo | (221) |
| Section 5 | Alopecia | (222) |
| Section 6 | Earyly Greying of Hair | (223) |
| Section 7 | Impetigo | (226) |
| Section 8 | Scleroderma | (227) |

## Chapter Seven
## Medicated Liquors for Nourishments and Longevity

| | | |
|---|---|---|
| Section 1 | Hypomnesis | (229) |
| Section 2 | Senile Lassitude in the Loin and Legs | (232) |
| Section 3 | Deficiency of Yang | (235) |
| Section 4 | Deficiency of Qi | (238) |
| Section 5 | Deficiency of Blood | (243) |
| Section 6 | Deficiency of Both Qi and Yin | (246) |
| Section 7 | Deficiency of Both Qi and Blood | (250) |
| Section 8 | Additional Prescriptions for Health Preserving | (255) |

# Chapter One
# Internal Diseases

## Section 1  Fever

    The temperature is a simple, objective and accurate indicator of a physiologic state. In general, an oral temperature above 37.2 degrees centigrade in a person at bed rest is regarded as probable indication of disease. Fever is classically described as intermittent, remittent, sustained, and relapsing. It accelerates many metabolic processes. In traditional Chinese medicine, fever is generally divided into two types: the sthenic-heat and asthenic-heat. The former is mainly caused by pathogenic factors, while the latter results from hyperactivity of yang due to impairment of vital energy, blood, and vital essence, or incoordination among the organs resulting in deficiency of yin. Feverish sensation and abnormal sensation of warmth are put under the same category of fever in traditional Chinese medicine. In fact, the temperatures of most sthenic cases are often normal.

    Since fever (sthenic type) ordinarily does little harm and imposes no great discomfort, antipyretic drugs are rarely essential to patient welfare and may obfuscate the effect of a specific therapeutic agent or of the natural course of the disease. There are situations, however, in which lowering of the body temperature is of vital importance; e.g., heat stroke, postoperative hyperthermia, delirium due to hyperpyrexia, epileptic seizures, or shock associated with fever and heart failure. Under these circumstances lowering the temperature is indicated. Sponging the body surface especially the forehead with alcohol is a highly effective mean for external cooling. Various management may be given to patients with fever according to different causes.

    The following recipes are effective for fever or for preventing the occurrence of fever as a presentation in some diseases.

**Recipe 1**
**Ingredients**
Pericarpium Zanthoxyli, 50 grains
Cacumen Platycladi Orientalis, 15 g
plain spirits, 500 ml

**Process**   The two drugs are pounded in a mortar and then are mixed with 500 ml of plain spirits in a bottle sealed airtightly for half one month.

**Directions**   The drink is warmed and taken 5-10 ml before breakfast every morning in the epidemic seasons of infectious respiratory and gastrointestinal diseases.

**Indications**   The drink is effective for preventing infectious diseases characterized by fever, headache, etc..

**Recipe** 2
**Ingredients**
Herba Lophatheri, 120 g

plain spirits, just the right amount

**Process**  Cut the fresh bamboo leaves into pieces and extract their juice; then add in plain spirits and mix them well.

**Directions**  The drink is taken 20 ml three times a day.

**Indications**  The drink is effective for infective fever caused by either bacteria or viruses.

**Recipe** 3
**Ingredients**
Anguilla Japonica, 500 g

millet wine, 500 ml

water, right amount

**Process**  Cut the sea eels open and remove its internal organs; add in 500 ml of millet wine and right amount of water and cook them over a slow fire until the fish is well-done. Salt and vinegar may be added if the patient likes.

**Directions**  Take the eels within two days.

**Indications**  The recipe has the effect of invigorating the asthenic organs and clearing away asthenic heat. So it should be given to patients with some kind of disease marked by mild fever, etc..

**Recipe** 4
**Ingredients**
Fructus Jujubae, 250 g

suet, 25 g

millet wine, 250 ml

**Process**  First decoct the Chinese date until it is softened; discharge water and add the suet and millet wine in, decoct them over a strong fire until the wine boils. Put them in a bottle and seal the bottle airtightly for 7 days.

**Directions**  Take 3-5 pieces of Chinese date twice daily.

**Indication**  Low-grade fever.

## Section 2 Headache

The term headache should encompass all aches and pains located in the head, but in common language its application is restricted to unpleasant sensations in the region of the cranial vault. Headache, along with fatigue, hunger, and thirst, represents the most frequent human discomforts. Medically speaking, its significance is often abstruse, for it may stand as a symptomatic expression of disease or of some minor tension or fatigue, incident to the affairs of the day. Fortunately, in most instances it reflects the latter, and only exceptionally does it warn of serious disease seated in intracranial structures. In traditional Chinese medicine, the head is the confluence of all yang-channels and the brain is known as the sea of marrow, both being closely related to the kidney essence. Headache may caused by either exogenous pathogens or internal injury. The following types of headache are caused by invasion of exogenous attack of pathogenic evils: acute headache involving the nape and back which is aggravated by exposure to wind or distending headache accompanied by flushed complexion and conjunctival congestion, and heaviness sensation in the head like being tightly bound, accompanied by chilliness and fever. Moderate intermittent headache running a long course usually pertains to pain caused by internal injury. It is mainly due to deficiency of the body.

The following recipes are generally effective for headache of asthenic type, which is caused by hypofunction of the vital energy, blood, and vital essence, or impairment of the organs.

**Recipe** 1

**Ingredients**

Semen Juglandis, 30 g

white sugar, 50 g

millet wine, 50 ml

**Process**  Pound the walnut kernel into a mash, mix it thoroughly with white sugar; put the mixture in a pot, add in 50 ml of millet wine and cook on a slow fire for 10 minutes.

**Directions**  Take it twice daily.

**Indication**  Headache as a presentation of postconcussional syndrome.

**Recipe** 2

**Ingredients**

pork brain, 2

Rhizoma Zingiberis Recens, right amount

millet wine, 100 ml

**Process**  Cut the ginger into pieces and extract their juice; put pork brain in a bowl, add one glass of ginger juice and 100 ml of millet wine in; steam them by putting the bowl in boiling water in a pot.

**Directions**  Take them all once other day.

**Indication**  Headache with a history of repeated attacks.

**Recipe** 3

**Ingredients**

Pseudosciaena Polyactis, right amount

millet wine, right amount

**Process**  Bake the air bladders of yellow croakers with their original property retained; grind them into fine powder.

**Directions**  Take a right amount of this powder twice a day.

**Indication**  Head-wind syndrome, a recurrent paroxysmal he adache caused by the attack of wind-cold or wind-heat evils or blood stasis and phlegm retention in the meridians of the head.

**Recipe** 4
**Ingredients**
Bulbus Allii Fistulosi, 50 g
air bladder of fish, 50 g
millet wine, 50 ml
salt, right amount
sesame oil, right amount

**Process**  Make soup with air bladders and scalli on stalk; after they are well-done, season the soup with sesame oil and salt.

**Directions**  Take the soup with millet wine.

**Indication**  Headache due to deficiency of vital energy.

**Recipe** 5
**Ingredients**
Aristichthys Nobilis, 1
Rhizoma Zingiberis Recens, 50 g
millet rice, 200 ml

**Process**  Cut the head of spotted silver carp into pieces, add the ginger and millet rice in, cook them with half a bowl of water in an earthenware pot.

**Directions**  After they have been well done, take the fish and soup warmly.

**Indication**  Migraine, a recurrent, intense headache usually confined to one side of the temporal region, occasional referring to the eye or accompanied with nausea, vomiting and visual disturbances; mostly due to attack of wind-evil to Gallbladder Meridian, or stagnation of phlegm-fire resulting from asthenia of the liver.

**Recipe** 6
**Ingredients**
Flos Chrysanthemi, 2000 g
Radix Rehmanniae, 1000 g
Radix Angelicae Sinensis, 500 g
Fructus Lycii, 500 g
rice, 3000 g

**Process**  Decoct the chrysanthemum flower, Chinese fox-glove root, Chinese angelica and barbary wolfberry fruit with right amount of water; remove the dregs from the decoction. Steam the rice until it is half-done. Dry the rice and then mix it with the decoction well; steam the mixture until it is well-done; add right amount of distiller's yeast in and put the mixture in an earthen jar, seal the jar airtightly. Preserve the temperature of the jar well. The fermentation is successful when the mixture tastes sweet.

**Directions**  Take three spoons of such drink with water twice daily.

**Indication**  Headache due to insufficiency of both liver and kidney-yin.

### Recipe 7
**Ingredients**
Rhizoma Ligustici Chuanxiong, 6 g
Radix Angelica Dahuricae, 6 g
polished glutinous rice, 60 ml

**Process**  Put the Szechwan lovage rhizome and Taiwan angelica root in a bowl and add the polished glutinous rice in; steam the mixture by putting the bowl in boiling water in a pot; remove the dregs from the decoction.

**Directions**  Take the decoction at bedtime daily.

**Indications**  Wind-headache syndrome and migraine.

### Recipe 8
**Ingredients**
Flos Chrysanthemi, 60 g
Fructus Lycii, 60 g
Shaoxing millet rice, right amount

**Process**  Soak the chrysanthemum flower and barbary wolfberry fruit in Shaoxing millet rice, seal the container and put it in a cool, dry place for 10 to 20 days; remove the dregs and add a right amount of honey in the tincture and stir the mixture equally. Store it up for future administration.

**Directions**  Take one glass of such drink twice daily.

**Indication**  Headache accompanied by dizziness.

### Recipe 9
**Ingredients**
Herba Asari, 3 g
Radix Adenophorae, 30 g
Fructus Viticis, 10 g
Rhizoma Ligustici Chuanxiong, 30 g
plain spirits, 300 ml

**Process**  Put the drugs in a pot, add 1000 ml of water in and then decoct them to make decoction until 700 ml of water is left; add 300 ml of plain spirits, mix them thoroughly for oral administration.

**Directions**  Take 30 ml of such drink three times daily. 7 days' administration consisted of one course of treatment.

**Indication**  Headache.

**Recipe** 10
**Ingredients**
sunflower seed, right amount
sunflower leaf, right amount
plain spirits, right amount
**Process**  Soak the ingredients in plain spirits, seal the container and put it in a cool, dry place for 12 hours; remove the dregs and store the extracts for future administration.
**Directions**  Take such drink 2-3 g, three times a day.
**Indication**  Headache due to influenza.

## Section 3 Common Cold and Influenza

The term "common cold" was invented to describe the coryzal syndrome before its diverse causes were known. It refers to illness characterized by nasal obstruction and discharge, sneezing, moderate sore throat, and mild constitutional reaction, usually without fever. Most respiratory viral infections may produce this picture. In adult and older children, two-thirds of cases of acute respiratory viral disease are caused by infection with rhinoviruses, respiratory syncytial virus, and coronaviruses. Herpesvirus causes disease usually localized to the pharynx and tonsils. The other viruses such as Coronaviruses, adenoviruses, while causing coryzal syndrome, also cause varying degree of involvement of the lower part of the respiratory tract, with additional symptoms. Influenza is an acute respiratory infection of specific viral etiology symbolized by sudden onset of headache, myalgia, fever, and prostration. The term "influenza" should be restricted to those cases with distinct epidemiologic or laboratory evidence of infection with influenza viruses. In traditional Chinese medicine, the term cold refers to the syndrome symptomized by headache, nasal obstruction, sneezing, nasal discharge, aversion to cold, fever, etc.. The syndrome is differentiated into several types according to distinctive manifestations. Common cold belongs to the categories of wind-cold and wind-heat, while influenza is considered to be involved in the prevalent epidemic pathogens.

**Recipe** 1
**Ingredients**
Flos Chrysanthemi, 60 g
Fructus Lycii, 60 g
millet wine, 200 ml
Mel, 20 g
**Process**  Soak barbary wolfberry fruit and chrysanthemum flower in 200 ml of millet wine, seal the container and put it in a cool, dry place for 10 to 20 days. Then add 20 g of honey in the tincture and stir equally for future administration.

**Directions**  Take the liquid 10 ml twice daily.

**Indication**  Common cold of wind-heat type marked by headache and mild fever.

### Recipe 2
**Ingredients**

red wine, 20 ml

egg, 1

**Process**  Heat the wine on slow fire, add in the egg, stop heating after stirring the mixture for one second.

**Directions**  Take the liquid before it cools.

**Indication**  Common cold.

### Recipe 3
**Ingredients**

grass carp, 1

mutton, 150 g

rice wine, 100 ml

Rhizoma Zingiberis, 25 g

**Process**  Cook the fish, mutton, ginger and rice wine in boiled water (right amount). Salt may be added in when required.

**Directions**  Take the meat and drink the soup while the food is hot in order to cause mild perspiration. Twice daily. Keep the patient away from wind and cold.

**Indication**  Common cold manifested by aversion to cold and headache.

### Recipe 4
**Ingredients**

litchi, 30 g

millet wine

**Process**  Cook the litchi in right amount of millet wine.

**Directions**  Take the fruit while it is hot.

**Indication**  Common cold of wind-cold type.

### Recipe 5
**Ingredients**

Semen Sesami Nigrum, 50 g

millet wine

**Process**  Bake the sesame and then grind into powder after it isdone.

**Directions**  Take it with millet wine of right amount to cause mild perspiration.

**Indication**  Common cold of wind-cold type.

**Recipe** 6
**Ingredients**
Bulbus Allii, 30 g
Semen Sojae Preparatum, 10 g
Rhizoma Zingiberis, 5 g
millet wine, 30 ml

**Process**  Decoct Chinese green onion, fermented soybean and ginger in 500 ml of water. After they are done, remove the dregs and add in 30 ml of millet wine.

**Directions**  Take the decoction when it is hot to cause perspiration.

**Indication**  Common cold of wind-cold type marked by headache, anhidrosis and restlessness.

**Recipe** 7
**Ingredients**
Bulbus Allii, 30 g
Rhizoma Zingiberis, 30 g
salt, 6 g
spirit, 30-50 ml

Pound the onion, ginger and salt until they become a paste. Add in 30-50 ml spirit and mix it well. Wrap the paste up with a piece of gauze.

**Directions**  Apply the mixture on the chest, back, soles and palms, and popliteal fossa. Ask the patient to sleep without anxiety. Perspiration usually occur 30 minutes after application.

**Indication**  Common cold of wind-cold type marked by fever andother general symptoms.

**Recipe** 8
**Ingredients**
Bulbus Allii, 20 g
spirit
millet

**Process**  Cook the onion and right amount of spirit and millet to make gruel.

**Directions**  Take the gruel when it is hot to cause sweat. Or take fresh onion with warm spirit.

**Indication**  Common cold of wind-cold type.

**Recipe** 9
**Ingredients**
Semen Sinapis Albae, 150 g
spirit, 250 ml

Wrap the mustard seed up with a piece of gauze, and cook it in 250 ml of spirit until it boils.

**Directions**  Compress the gauze to the skin of the neck and nape when the gauze is hot. Apply compress therapy twice to four times daily. Take 5 ml of spirit twice to three times daily in the mean time.

**Indication**  Used for prevention of the attack of influenza. Contraindicated for cases who have histories of allergic dermatitis.

**Recipe** 10
**Ingredients**
Radix Sophorae Flavescentis, 3 g
Radix Platycodi, 1 g
spirit, 250 ml

**Process** Pound the balloonflower root and lightyellow sophora root into powder and wrap up with a piece of gauze. Cook the powder in 250 ml of spirit on slow fire for 10 minutes. After it is done, seal the powder and spirit up in a bottle for later use.

**Directions and Indication**  Apply the tincture to the nares twice to four times daily for prevention of influenza during epidemic seasons.

**Recipe** 11
**Ingredients**
Pericarpium Zanthoxyli, 50 grains
Cacumen Platycladi Orientalis, 15 g
spirit, 500 ml

**Process**  Pound the bunge pricklyash peel and oriental arborvitae leafytwigs into powder and wrap up along with 500 ml of spirit in a clean bottle for half one month.

**Directions**  Take 5-10 ml of the tincture before breakfast once daily.

**Indication**  Applied for prevention of influenza and other respiratory disorders in epidemic seasons.

## Section 4  Cough

Cough is one of the most frequent cardiorespiratory symptoms. It is an eruptive expiration which provides a way of clearing the tracheobronchial tree of secretions and foreign bodies. Cough is produced by inflammatory, mechanical, chemical, and thermal stimulation of the cough receptors. Inflammatory stimuli are initiated by edema and hyperemia of the respiratory mucous membranes, and by irritation from exudative processes. Such stimuli may arise either in the airways or in the alveoli. Mechanical stimuli are produced by inhalation of particulate matter, such as dust particles, and by compression of the air passages and pressure or tension upon these structures. Lesions associated with airway compression may be either extramural or intramural in type. Pressure or tension upon the air passages is usually produced by lesions associated with a decrease in pulmonary compliance. Specific causes include acute and chronic interstitial fibrosis, pulmonary edema, and atelectasis, etc.. Chemical stimuli may result from inhalation of irritant gases, including cigarette smoke and chemical fumes.

Thermal stimuli may produced by inhalation of either very hot or cold air. In traditional Chinese medicine, cough refers to a syndrome manifested mainly by cough. Cough is presentation of impairment of purifying and descending function of the lung leading to adverse rising of lung-qi. There are generally two types in the clinic: the exopathogenic and endopathogenic types. The former is mainly due to invasion of wind-cold or wind-heat affecting the lung and defensive qi of the body, leading to dysfunction of the lung in descending and dispersing. The latter is mostly due to repeated attacks of cough, leading to chronic damage of lung-qi. Deficiency of lung-qi may affects the spleen and leads to deficiency of spleen-qi, which will cause the occurring of internal dampness and phlegm. The dampness and phlegm may further affect the lung. On the other hand, stagnation of liver-qi turning into heat-evil may also result in the endopathogenic cough when it ascends to the lung and leads to insufficiency of lung fluid.

The subsequent prescriptions are effective for cough of various types.

**Recipe** 1
**Ingredients**
lard, 120 g
sesame oil, 120 g
Mel, 120 g
tea powder, 120 g
spirit, 120 ml

**Process**　Soak the lard, sesame oil, honey and tea powder in the spirit in an earthen jar, cover the lid, heat the mixture until it boils. After the mixture condenses to solid, store it up for future administration.

**Directions**　Take right amount of condensation along with tea once daily.

**Indication**　Cough due to retention of cold evil.

**Recipe** 2
**Ingredients**
skin of soya-bean milk
mellow win

**Process**　Parch the skin of soya-bean milk with its nature retained. Then grind the parched skin into powder for later use.

**Directions**　Take 40-50 g of powder with warm old wine once daily.

**Indication**　Cough of cold type.

**Recipe** 3
**Ingredients**
Semen Juglandis, 1
millet wine, 15 ml

**Process**　Bake the walnut kernel over slow fire. Then grind it into powder for later use.

**Directions** Take the powder with millet wine twice daily.
**Indication** Cough worsened by wind-cold evil.

### Recipe 4
**Ingredients**
Semen Juglandis, 100 g
white sugar, 500 g
millet wine, 150 ml
**Process** Pound the walnut to pieces and then cook it along with white sugar in millet wine over a medium fire until it boils. Then heat it over a slow fire for 10 minutes.
**Directions** Take the kernel once or twice daily. One course consists of 3 to 10 days.
**Indication** Cough of asthenic type due to deficiency of kidney-essence and lack of body fluid.

### Recipe 5
**Ingredients**
Pancreas of sheep, 3
Fructus Jujubae, 300 g
spirit, 1000 ml
**Process** Soak the pancreata and jujubes in 1000 ml of spirit, seal the container and put it in a cool, dry place for 7 days. Shake the container once daily during soaking. Filter the mixture and store the extracts up for future administration.
**Directions** Drink right amount of the extracts once daily.
**Indication** Chronic cough.

### Recipe 6
**Ingredients**
Fructus Perillae, 60 g
Semen Armeniacae Amarum, 15 g
Pericarpium Trichosanthis, 15 g
Bulbus Fritillariae Unibracteatae, 15 g
Rhizoma Pinelliae, 15 g
Fructus Aurantii, 15 g
Radix Stemonae, 15 g
Radix Platycodi, 15 g
Cortex Mori Radicis, 15 g
Folium Eriobotryae, 15 g
Poria, 15 g
Pericarpium Citri Reticulatae, 30 g
Rhizoma Zingiberis, 30 g
Herba Asari Heterotropoidedis, 7.5 g

Fructus Amomi Rotundus, 7.5 g
Fructus Schisandrae Chinensis, 7.5 g
Radix Glycyrrhizae, 1.5 g
spirit, 2500 ml

**Process**  Pound the above ingredients (except spirit) into powder. Fill a gauze bag with the powder and then soak it in 2500 ml of plain spirits and seal the container. Shake it once other day during soaking. 12 days later, open the container and filter the tincture to remove the dregs.

**Directions**  30 to 50 ml twice daily.

**Indication**  Cough of wind-cold type characterized by cough with dyspnea, nasal obstruction and discharge, itching sensation in the throat, thin whitish sputum, headache and fever, aversion to cold or wind.

### Recipe 7
**Ingredients**
Fructus Perillae, 60 g
millet wine, 2500 ml

**Process**  Stir-fry the perilla fruit over a slow fire and then fill them in a gauze bag, fasten its mouth and soak it in millet wine, seal the container and put it in a cool, dry place for 7 days. Shake the container once daily during soaking. Filter the tincture and store it up for future administration.

**Directions**  Drink the tincture 10 ml once daily.

**Indication**  Cough due to retention of phlegm and abnormal rising of lung qi. Contraindicated for cough of heat type.

### Recipe 8
**Ingredients**
azalea, 15 g
spirit, 500 ml

**Process**  Cut the dried azalea into pieces, Soak them in the spirit and seal the container, put it in a cool, dry place for 5 days. Shake the container once daily during soaking. Filter the tincture and store it up for future administration.

**Directions**  Take 20 ml twice daily.

**Indications**  Cough due to phlegm retention and wind-heat, dyspnea, etc..

### Recipe 9
**Ingredients**
Cortex Mori Radicis, 150 g
Rhizoma Zingiberis, 9 g
Fructus Evodiae, 15 g
spirit 1000 ml

**Process**  Cook mulberry bark, fresh ginger and medicinal evodia fruit along with 500 ml of water and 1000 ml of spirit over a slow fire until there is 1000 ml of the decoction remained. Remove the dregs for later use.

**Directions**   Take 30 ml twice daily.

**Indications**   Cough with dyspnea, distention of the chest, vomiting of watery vomitus.

## Recipe 10
**Ingredients**
Cortex Mori Radicis, 200 g
rice wine, 1000 ml

**Process**   Cut mulberry bark into pieces, soak them in rice wine and seal the container for 7 days. Keep the container from heat and shake the container once daily during soaking. Filter the tincture and store it up for future administration.

**Directions**   Take 15 to 20 ml three time daily.

**Indication**   Cough due to lung heat marked by cough, profuse sputum of yellowish color, dyspnea, etc..

## Recipe 11
**Ingredients**
Semen Lepidii, 200 g
rice wine, 1000 ml

**Process**   Bake pepperweed seed over a slow fire then grind them into powder. Fill a gauze bag with the powder and soak it in rice wine and seal the container, put it in a cool, dry place for 7 days. Shake the container once daily during soaking. Filter the tincture and store it up for future administration.

**Directions**   Take 20 ml twice daily.

**Indications**   Cough with dyspnea due to abnormal rising of lung qi, cough due to phlegm retention, edema, etc..

## Recipe 12
**Ingredients**
Radix Stemonae, 100 g
spirit, 1000 ml

**Process**   Cut tubers of stemona root into pieces. Bake them over a slow fire for a few seconds. Soak the pieces in 1000 ml of spirit and seal the container, put it in a cool, dry place for 7 days. Shake the container once daily during soaking. Filter the tincture and store it up for future administration.

**Directions**   20 ml three times daily. Avoid acrid or pungent food and seafood.

**Indications**   Acute and chronic cough.

## Recipe 13

**Ingredients**

Mel, 250 g

Saccharum Granorum, 250 g

Rhizoma Zingiberis, 500 g

Radix Stemonae, 500 g

Fructus Jujubae, 100 g

Semen Armeniacae Amarum, 100 g

Pericarpium Citri Reticulatae, 60 g

**Process**  Extract fresh ginger, tubers of stemon a root to get juice and pound jujubes and apricot seed into mash. Grind tangerine peel into powder. Then decoct the mash of apricot seed and juice of tuber stemona root along with 1000 ml of water over a medium fire until 500 ml of water remained. Remove the dregs and add honey, juice of ginger, malt extract, mash of jujubes and powder of tangerine peel in. Decoct the mixture over a slow fire until the mixture changes into semifluid.

**Directions**  Take the mixture 10 to 20 g along with warm wine three times daily.

**Indications**  Cough due to deficiency of lung qi and attack of wind-cold evil marked by cough with dyspnea, aversion to cold and fever, etc..

**Recipe 14**

**Ingredients**

Ganoderma Lucidum, 50 g

Radix Ginseng, 20 g

crystal sugar, 500 g

spirit, 1500 ml

**Process**  Cut lucid ganoderma and ginseng into thin slices. Fill the dried slices along with crystal sugar in a clean gauze bag. Soak it in 1500 ml of spirit and seal the container, put it in a cool, dry place for 10 days. Shake the container once daily during soaking. Filter the tincture and store it up for future administration.

**Directions**  Take the tincture 15 to 20 ml twice daily.

**Indications**  Chronic cough due to consumption, profuse sputum, dyspnea due to deficiency of lung qi, indigestion, insomnia.

**Recipe 15**

**Ingredients**

Pericarpium Citri Reticulatae, 30 g

spirit, 500 ml

**Process**  Soak red tangerine peel in 500 ml of spirit and seal the container, put it in a cool, dry place for 7 days. Shake the container once daily during soaking. Filter the tincture and store it up for future administration.

**Directions**  Take 5 ml before sleep.

**Indication**  Repeated cough worsened by cold evil.

**Recipe** 16
**Ingredients**
Retinervus Luffae Fructus
Fructus Jujubae
spirit
**Process**  Parch vegetable sponge of luffa with its nature retained. Then grind the parched vegetable sponge into powder. Mix the powder and jujubes to make pills. The size of the pill is similar to that of a jujube.
**Directions**  Take one pill twice daily.
**Indications**  Cough with dyspnea due to retention of phlegm.

**Recipe** 17
**Ingredients**
Pericarpium Citri Reticulatae
spirit
**Process**  Cut fresh tangerine peel into slices and then soak them in right amount of spirit, seal the container and put it in a cool, dry place for three days. Shake the container once daily during soaking. Filter the tincture and store it up for future administration.
**Directions**  Drink 10 ml twice daily.
**Indication**  Cough due to lung heat.

**Recipe** 18
**Ingredients**
Rhizoma Bletillae, 10 g
Lungs of a pig
spirit
**Process**  Cook the lungs and bletilla tubers in right amount of spirit until it boils.
**Directions**  Take the lungs and drink the soup.
**Indications**  Cough accompanied by chest pain and purulent sputum.

**Recipe** 19
**Ingredients**
Folium Mori, 500 g
millet wine
**Process**  Grind mulberry leaves into powder.
**Directions**  Take 4 to 5 g of the powder along with right amount of millet wine twice daily.
**Indications**  Cough due to consumption, yellowish sputum or purulent sputum.

**Recipe** 20

**Ingredients**
Gecko, 1
Radix Codonopsis Pilosulae, 30 g
Radix Astragali, 30 g
rice wine, 1500 ml
**Process** Soak the gecko, pilose Asiabell root and milkvetch root in 1500 ml of rice wine, put it in a cool, dry place for lateruse.
**Directions** Drink 10-20 ml once daily.
**Indications** Cough with dyspnea due to deficiency of lung qi and kidney qi.

**Recipe** 21
**Ingredients**
Rhopilema, 500 g
Bulbus Heleocharis Tuberosae, 100
spirit, 1500 ml
**Process** Soak the jellyfish and water chestnut in 1500 ml of spirit, seal the container and put it in a cool, dry place for 7 days. Shake the container once daily during soaking. Filter the tincture and store it up for future administration.
**Directions** Take 7 water chestnuts before breakfast.
**Indications** Cough due to phlegm and heat evil, subcutaneousnodule.

## Section 5 Pulmonary Abscess

A pulmonary abscess is a necrotic area of lung parenchyma containing purulent material. The pathogenesis of infectious lung abscesses is nearly identical to that of pneumonia. Most arise from the aspiration of naso-or oropharyngeal contents. The development of a lung abscess depends upon the infecting organism's ability to cause necrosis of lung tissue. Less frequently, abscesses arise from hematogenous spread of organisms to the lung. This way occur during bacteremia originating from a distant site of infection or as a result of septic emboli either from right-sided endocarditis or from septic thrombophlebitis associated with infections in the extremities or the abdominal cavity.

**Recipe** 1
**Ingredients**
Rhizoma Bletillae, 30 g
pork lungs, one set
spirits, right amount
**Process** Wash pork lungs clean. Cook the lungs and common bletilla tubers with a right amount of spirits until they are done.

**Directions**  Take the lungs and drink the soup.
**Indication**  Pulmonary abscess.

**Recipe 2**
**Ingredients**
Rhizoma Fagopyri Cymosi, 60 g
millet wine, 100 ml

**Process**  Steam the cymose buckwheat rhizome along with 100 ml of millet wine in a container in boiling water for 45 minutes. Then remove the dregs for later use.
**Directions**  Take 20 ml of the tincture twice daily.
**Indication**  Pulmonary abscess.

**Recipe 3**
**Ingredients**
Fructus Luffae
millet wine

**Process**  Burn the towel gourds into charcoal with their nature retained. Grind the parched gourds into fine powder.
**Directions**  Take 10 g of the powder with a right amount of warm wine, twice daily.
**Indication**  Pulmonary abscess.

## Section 6 Asthma

Asthma is disease of airways that is typified by increased responsiveness of the tracheobronchial tree to a multiplicity of stimuli. Asthma is manifested physiologically by a sweeping narrowing of the air passages which may be relieved spontaneously or as a result of therapy. Asthma is manifested clinically by paroxysms of dyspnea, cough, and wheezing. It is an episodic disease, acute exacerbations being interspersed with symptom-free periods. Typically, most attacks are short-lived, lasting minutes to hours, and after them the patient seems to recover completely clinically. Allergic asthma is often associated with a personal and/or family history of allergic diseases; positive wheal-and-flare skin reactions to intradermal injection of extracts of airborne antigens; increased levels of IgE in the serum; and/or positive response to provocation tests involving the inhalation of specific antigen. Immunologic mechanisms appear to be causally related to the development of asthma in 25 to 35 percent of all cases. Allergic asthma is usually seasonal, and it is most often observed in children and young adults. A non-seasonal form may result from allergy to feathers, animal danders, molds, and other antigens present continuously in the environment. In traditional Chinese medicine, it belongs to "xiao chuan". At the stage of attack, there are two types of syndromes, namely, asthma of cold type and asthma of heat type. The former is characterized by rapid breathing, wheezing sound in the throat, chocking sensation in the chest much like asphyxia, dim and blackish complexion, cold extremities, non-thirst or thirst but desire for hot drink, easy to be attacked in cold weather or when taken with cold, white and slippery fur, and tense or floating and tense pulse. Asthma of heat type is symptomized by dyspnea and raucous breathing, thunderous rale in the throat, fits of irritated cough, cough with yellow, ropy and thick phlegm, difficult expectoration, vexation, restlessness, flushed face, bitter taste, thirst and desire for drink, perspiration, or accompanied with fever, red tongue with yellowish and greasy fur, slippery rapid pulse. The following prescriptions based on differential diagnosis can be selected and used in light of its clinical manifestations.

**Recipe 1**
**Ingredients**
Cordyceps, 20 g
spirit, 100 g
**Process** Grind the Chinese caterpillar fungus into powder and then soak in the spirit and seal the container, put it in a cool, dry place for 15 days. Shake the container once daily during soaking. Filter the tincture and store it up for future administration.
**Directions** Take 10-15 ml once daily.
**Indications** Emission and impotency, cough due to consumption, hemoptysis, night sweat, tuberculosis, chronic cough with dyspnea.

**Recipe 2**
**Ingredients**
Semen Sesami Nigrum, 25 g
Semen Juglandis, 25 g
spirit, 500 ml
**Process** Soak the sesame and walnut kernel in the spirit and seal the container, put it in a cool, dry place for 15 days. Shake the container once daily during soaking. Filter the tincture and store it up for future administration.
**Directions** 15-20 g twice daily.
**Indications** Cough due to deficiency of kidney qi, lumbago and weakness of the lower extremities, emission and impotency, constipation.

**Recipe 3**
**Ingredients**
Semen Juglandis, 50 g
white sugar, 500 g
plain spirits, 600 ml
**Process** Remove the walnut shells and pound the kernels into pieces. Soak the kernels in plain spirit and seal the container, put it in a cool, dry place for 15 days. Shake the container once daily during soaking. Filter the tincture and add white sugar in, stir the mixture equally, store it up for fu-

ture administration.

**Directions**  Take 15 ml three times daily.

**Indications**  Cough due to deficiency of kidney qi, lumbago and weakness of the lower extremities, emission and impotency, constipation.

### Recipe 4
**Ingredients**
Rhizoma Zingiberis, 30 g
Semen Sinapis Albae, 10 g
spirit

**Process**  Cut the ginger into thin slices and pound them to obtain juice. Grind the white mustard seed along with the juice of ginger and right amount of spirit into paste. Apply the paste on the points Feishu(BL13), Dazhui(DU14), and Danzhong(RN17). Rub the points for 10 minutes.

**Directions**  Three times daily.

**Indication**  Bronchial asthma.

### Recipe 5
**Ingredients**
Fructus Trichosanthis, 12 g
Bulbus Allii Macrostemi, 9 g
spirit

**Process**  Decoct snakegourd fruit and macrostem onion along with right amount of spirit over a slow fire until the decoction boils.

**Directions**  Take the decoction 5 ml 3 times daily.

**Indications**  Asthma, cough with dyspnea.

### Recipe 6
**Ingredients**
Fructus Evodiae, 30 g
Semen Impatientis, 60 g
wheat flour
rice wine

**Process**  Grind garden balsam seed and medicinal evodia fruit into powder and mix cakes with right amount of wheat flour and rice wine. Paste the cakes up to the back of the patient.

**Directions**  Three times daily.

**Indication**  Asthma due to retention of phlegm.

# Section 7 Dyspepsia

Dyspepsia or indigestion refers to disordered digestion usually applied to pain or discomfort in the lower chest or abdomen after eating and is sometimes accompanied by nausea or vomiting. It is a term frequently used by patients to describe a multitude of symptoms generally appreciated as distress associated with the intake of food. Indigestion may occur as a result of disease of the gastrointestinal tract or is associated with pathologic states in other organ systems. In traditional Chinese medicine, it is considered to be concerned with deficiency of spleen and stomach, disharmony between spleen and stomach, stagnation of liver qi affecting the spleen or stomach, etc..

**Recipe** 1
**Ingredients**
Fructus Tsaoko, 10 g
spirit, 250 ml
Fructus Crataegi, 5 g
**Process**  Soak tsaoko cardamon and hawthorn fruit in spirit and seal the container, put it in a cool, dry place for 7 to 10 days. Shake the container once daily during soaking. Filter the tincture and store it up for future administration.
**Directions**  Take 10-15 ml twice daily.
**Indications**  Indigestion, distending pain in the epigastric region, regurgitation of food from stomach.

**Recipe** 2
**Ingredients**
Rhizoma Atractylodis Macrocephalae, 60 g
Poria, 60 g
Flos Chrysanthemi, 60 g
Folium Lonicerae, 40 g
old wine, 1500 ml
**Process**  Pound bighead atractylodes rhizome, poria and chrysanthemum flowers into pieces and cut honey-suckle leaves into thin stripes. Fill them in a gauze bag, soak it in old wine and seal the container, put it in a cool, dry place for 7 days. Shake the container once daily during soaking. Filter the tincture and add 1000 ml of water in, store it up for future administration.
**Directions**  Take 10 to 15 ml twice daily.
**Indications**  Retention of dampness due to deficiency of spleen marked by distention of the epigastric region, palpitation, blurring of vision, heavy sensation of the waist and lower extremities.

**Recipe** 3
**Ingredients**
Fructus Amomi, 60 g
millet wine, 500 g

**Process**  Cook amomum fruit and grind them into powder. Fill in a gauze bag in millet wine with the container sealed for 3 to 5 days.

**Directions**  Take 15 ml warmly, three times daily.

**Indications**  Distention of the chest and abdomen, anorexia, indigestion, hernia, nausea and vomiting, stomachache, diarrhea, dysentery.

**Recipe** 4
**Ingredients**
Fructus Citri Sarcodactylis, 30 g
spirits, 1000 ml

**Process**  Cut finger citron into slices and soak them in spirit with the container sealed, put it in a cool, dry place for 10 days. Shake the container once daily during soaking. Filter the tincture and store it up for future administration.

**Directions**  Take 15 ml twice daily.

**Indications**  Stagnation of liver qi resulting in stagnation of spleen qi and stomach qi manifested by depressed emotion, anorexia, distention of the chest and hypochondria, nausea, vomiting, cough with abundant sputum.

**Recipe** 5
**Ingredients**
fresh roses, 350 g
crystal sugar, 200 g
spirits, 1500 g

**Process**  Pound crystal sugar into powder. Soak roses and crystal sugar in spirit and seal the container, put it in a cool, dry place for 40 days. Shake the container once daily during soaking. Filter the tincture and store it up for future administration.

**Directions**  Take 15 to 20 ml twice daily.

**Indications**  Incoordination between liver and stomach marked by indigestion, distending pain or colic in the epigastric region and hypochondria, frequent eructation, anorexia.

**Recipe** 6
**Ingredients**
Semen Oryzae cum Monasco, 15 g
Fructus Amomi, 15 g
Pericarpium Citri Reticulatae, 7.5 g
Pericarpium Citri Reticulatae Viride, 7.5 g

Radix Angelicae Sinensis, 7.5 g

Flos Caryophylli, 7.5 g

Fructus Amomi Rotundus, 7.5 g

Cortex Magnoliae Officinalis, 3 g

Fructus Gardeniae, 3 g

Fructus Hordei Germinatus, 3 g

Fructus Aurantii, 3 g

Herba Agastachis, 4.5 g

Radix Aucklandiae, 1.5 g

crystal sugar, 500 g

spirit, 4000 g

**Process** Fill the above ingredients except crystal sugar and spirit in a gauze bag and soak it in spirit, cover the lid of the container. Steam the container in boiling water in a food steamer for 2 hours. After it cools, remove the dregs and add crystal sugar in, stir the mixture equally for future administration.

**Directions** Take 15 to 20 ml twice daily.

**Indications** Stagnation of liver qi and deficiency of spleen qi marked by indigestion, distention of the chest and abdomen, anorexia, hiccup, belching.

**Recipe** 7
**Ingredients**
Rhizoma Cyperi, 30 g

spirit, 500 ml

**Process** Wash nutgrass flatsedge rhizome clean and cut into slices. Soak them in spirit and seal the container, put it in a cool, dry place for 7 to 10 days.

**Directions** Take 15 ml three times daily.

**Indications** Indigestion, hypochondriac pain due to stagnation of liver qi, abdominal pain during menstruation, distending pain in the epigastric region.

**Recipe** 8
**Ingredients**
Pericarpium Citri Reticulatae, 50 g

haw wine, 1000 ml

spirit, 500 ml

**Process** Cut tangerine peel into pieces and soak them in spirit with the container sealed, put it in a cool, dry place for 7 days. Remove the dregs and mix the tincture with haw wine equally, then store it up for future administration.

**Directions** Take 30 ml twice daily.

**Indications** Indigestion, anorexia, fullness sensation of the stomach, distention of the epigastric region.

**Recipe** 9
**Ingredients**
Fructus Crataegi, 250 g
Arillus Longan, 250 g
Fructus Jujubae, 30 g
brown sugar, 30 g
rice wine, 1000 ml
**Process**  Wash hawthorn fruit, longans and jujubes clean, Dry them and pound into powder. Soak the powder and brown sugar in rice wine and seal the container, put it in a cool, dry place for 10 days. Shake the container once daily during soaking. Filter the tincture and store it up for future administration.
**Directions**  Take 15 ml twice daily.
**Indications**  Incoordination between spleen and stomach manifested by distention of the epigastric region, indigestion, sallow face.

**Recipe** 10
**Ingredients**
beer
**Directions**  Drink 300 ml of beer half one hour after lunch and before sleep. One course consisting of 30 days.
**Indication**  Indigestion.

**Recipe** 11
**Ingredients**
red bayberry, 500 g
spirit, 1000 ml
**Process**  Wash bayberries clean and dry them. Soak them in spirit and seal the container, put it in a cool, dry place for 3 months. Shake the container once daily during soaking. Filter the tincture and store it up for future administration.
**Directions**  Take 15 ml twice daily.
**Indication**  Indigestion.

**Recipe** 12
**Ingredients**
Fructus Tsaoko, 10 g
spirit, 250 ml
**Process**  Soak tsaoko cardamon in spirit and seal the container, put it in a cool, dry place for 7 days. Shake the container once daily during soaking. Filter the tincture and store it up for future administration. **Directions**  Take 10 ml once daily.

**Indication**  Indigestion.

**Recipe** 13
**Ingredients**
Fructus Amomi, 30 g
spirit, 500 ml
**Process**  Pound amomum fruit into pieces and fill them in a clean gauze bag. Soak the bag in spirit and seal the container, put it in a cool, dry place for 7 days. Shake the container once daily during soaking. Filter the tincture and store it up for future administration.
**Directions**  Take 10 ml after meals.
**Indication**  Indigestion.

**Recipe** 14
**Ingredients**
Pericarpium Citri Reticulatae, 50 g
spirit, 500 g
**Process**  Soak tangerine peel in spirit and seal the container, put it in a cool, dry place for 7 days. Shake the container once daily during soaking. Filter the tincture and store it up for future administration.
**Directions**  Take 15 ml once daily.
**Indication**  Indigestion.

**Recipe** 15
**Ingredients**
green plum, 30 g
spirit, 500 g
**Process**  Soak green plums in spirit and seal the container, put it in a cool, dry place for 7 days. Shake the container once daily during soaking. Filter the tincture and store it up for future administration.
**Directions**  Take 15 ml once daily.
**Indications**  Indigestion, anoréxia, diarrhea.

**Recipe** 16
**Ingredients**
Radix Aucklandiae, 9 g
Flos Caryophylli, 6 g
Lignum Santali, 6 g
Radix Rubiae, 60 g
Fructus Amomi, 15 g
Semen Oryzae cum Monasco, 30 g

Mel, right amount

spirit, 500 ml

**Process**  Grind costus root, cloves, sandalwood, rubia root, amomum fruit and medicated leaven into fine powder. Mix it with honey to make pills. Each weighs about 9 g. Soak one pill in 500 ml of spirit, seal the container and put it in a cool, dry place for 7 days. Shake the container once daily during soaking. Filter the tincture and store it up for future administration.

**Directions**  Take 15 ml twice daily.

**Indications**  Indigestion, anorexia, distention of the epigastric region, belching, hiccup.

## Section 8 Anorexia

Anorexia, or loss of the desire to eat, is a prominent symptom in a wide variety of intestinal and extraintestinal disorders. It must be clearly differentiated from satiety and from specific food intolerance. Anorexia is commonly seen in diseases of the gastrointestinal tract and liver. For example, it may precede the appearance of jaundice in hepatitis, or it may be a prominent symptom in gastric carcinoma. In the setting of intestinal disease, anorexia should be clearly differentiated from sitophobia, or fear of eating because of subsequent or associated discomfort. In such circumstances, appetite may persist, but the ingestion of food is curtailed nonetheless. Anorexia may also be a prominent feature of severe extraintestinal diseases. For example, anorexia may be profound in severe congestive heart failure and is often associated with cardiac glycoside intoxication. It may be a major symptom in patients with uremia, pulmonary failure, and various endocrinopathies. Anorexia also often accompanies psychogenic disturbances, such as anxiety or depression. The subsequent prescriptions are effective for relieving the symptom due to intestinal diseases.

**Recipe** 1

**Ingredients**

green plum, 30 g

millet wine, 100 ml

**Process**  Soak green plums in millet wine and cover the lid of the container. Steam the container in boiling water for 20 minutes. After it cools, filter the decoction and store it up for future administration.

**Directions**  Take 10 ml warmly, twice daily.

**Indication**  Poor appetite.

**Recipe** 2

**Ingredients**

Rhizoma Cyperi, 60 g

spirit, 250 ml

water, 250 ml

**Process**  Wash nutgrass flatsedge rhizome clean and cut into pieces. Soak them in water and spirit and seal the container, put it in a cool, dry place for 3 to 5 days. Shake the container once daily during soaking. Filter the tincture and store it up for future administration.

**Directions**  Take 10 ml three times daily.

**Indication**  Poor appetite.

**Recipe** 3

**Ingredients**

water chestnut

spirit

**Process**  Wash fresh water chestnuts clean and soak them in spirit with the container sealed, put it in a cool, dry place for 30 days. Shake the container once daily during soaking. Filter the tincture and store it up for future administration.

**Directions**  Take 3 to 7 water chestnuts once daily. 5 days consisted of one course of treatment.

**Indications**  Anorexia, dry stools.

## Section 9 Vomiting

Vomiting refers to the forceful oral expulsion of gastric contents. It is conveniently considered together with nausea. Nausea often precedes or accompanies vomiting. It is usually associated with diminished functional activity of the stomach and alterations of the motility of the duodenum and small intestine. Following a period of nausea and a brief interval of retching, a sequence of involuntary visceral and somatic motor events occurs, resulting in vomiting. Nausea and vomiting are common manifestations of organic and functional disorders. Many acute abdominal emergencies which lead to the " surgical abdomen" are associated with nausea and vomiting. Notably, vomiting may be seen with inflammation of a viscus as in acute appendicitis or acute cholecystitis, obstruction of the intestine, or acute peritonitis. In many disorders involving chronic indigestion nausea and vomiting may be prominent. Acute systemic infections with fever, especially in young children, are frequently accompanied by vomiting and often by severe diarrhea. Central nervous system disorders which lead to increased intracranial pressure may be accompanied by vomiting. Severe nausea and vomiting may be present in acute myocardial infarction, especially of the posterior wall of the heart. They may also be seen in congestive heart failure. Several endocrinologic disorders are commonly accompanied by nausea and vomiting. And side effects of many drugs and chemical include nausea and vomiting. Vomiting may occur as part of any emotional upset on a transitory basis or more persistently as part of a psychic disturbance.

In traditional Chinese medicine, vomiting is considered to be concerned with the invasion of exogenous pathogenic factors such as wind, cold, summer-heat and dampness into the stomach along the Stomach Meridian. It leads to derangement of stomach qi so that the food substance and gastric fluid are cast up together with the abnormal ascending of gastric qi. Over intake of cold or raw food, or intake of sour food by mistake can cause food retention in the stomach and difficulty in the descending of stomach qi. Emotional depression or sudden emotional upset can cause liver qi to attack the stomach so that food substance reverses along with the abnormal ascending of gastric qi. Constitutional deficiency of the spleen and stomach or impairment of the spleen and stomach after illness cause the inactive yang of the middle jiao and poor transformation and transportation in which there will be retention of food and gastric fluid and stomach may lead to the poor moistening and descending function of the stomach.

### Recipe 1
**Ingredients**
red bayberry
spirit

**Process** Soak right amount of red bayberries in spirits, seal the container and put it in a cool, dry place for 7 days. Shake the container once daily during soaking. Filter the tincture and store it up for future administration.

**Directions** Take 1 or 2 red bayberries twice or three times daily.

**Indication** Vomiting.

### Recipe 2
**Ingredients**
fresh ginger juice, 5 ml
grape wine, 20 ml

**Process** Add fresh ginger juice in grape wine and shake the container frequently.

**Directions** Take the mixture daily.

**Indication** Vomiting.

### Recipe 3
**Ingredients**
crucian carp, 1
millet wine

**Process** Pound crucian carp to get juice.

**Directions** Take the juice along with right amount of millet wine.

**Indication** Vomiting due to deficiency of both spleen and stomach.

### Recipe 4
**Ingredients**
dried persimmon
millet wine

**Process**  Parch right amount of dried persimmons with their nature retained. Then grind the parched persimmon into powder.

**Directions**  Take 6 g of the powder with right amount of millet wine twice daily.

**Indications**  Vomiting and regurgitation.

### Recipe 5
**Ingredients**

Corneum Gigeriae Galli, 30 g

spirit

**Process**  Parch chicken's gizzard-skin with its nature retained. Grind the parched gizzard-skin into powder.

**Directions**  Take 3 g of the powder with right amount of spirit twice daily.

**Indication**  Vomiting and regurgitation.

### Recipe 6
**Ingredients**

Folium Perillae, 6 g

Pericarpium Citri Reticulatae, 6 g

spirit, 6 ml

**Process**  Decoct dried perilla leaves and tangerine peel along with spirit over strong fire until they are done.

**Directions**  Take the decoction daily.

**Indication**  Vomiting due to cold evil attack the stomach.

### Recipe 7
**Ingredients**

millet wine, 50 ml

Flos Caryophylli, 2 grains

**Process**  Soak cloves in millet wine in a container with the lid covered. Steam the container in boiling water for 10 minutes. After it cools, filter the decoction and store it up for future administration.

**Directions**  Take the wine when it is warm.

**Indications**  Vomiting and diarrhea due to cold evil.

### Recipe 8
**Ingredients**

cane sugar

**Process**  Cut cane sugar into pieces and extract their juice.

**Directions**  Take 400 ml of the juice.

**Indication**  Vomiting due to overdrunk.

**Recipe** 9
**Ingredients**
Gypsum Fibrosum, 8 g
salt, 20 g
Mel, 10 g
spirit

**Process**  Grind gypsum and salt into fine powder. Add honey and spirit in and mix them to get medicinal extract.

**Directions**  Apply the extract on Quepen(ST12).

**Indication**  Vomiting.

**Recipe** 10
**Ingredients**
Pericarpium Citri Reticulatae, 500 g
fructose (15%)
spirit 1300 ml

**Process**  Wash tangerine peel clean and cut into pieces. Parch them with their nature retained. Grind the parched peel into fine powder. Soak the powder in spirit for 2 minutes. Filter the mixture twice. Add right amount of fructose in and stir the mixture equally.

**Directions**  Take 15 ml twice daily.

**Indications**  Stagnation of spleen qi and stomach qi manifested by indigestion, distending pain in the epigastric region, nausea, vomiting

**Recipe** 11
**Ingredients**
Rhizoma Zingiberis, 100 g
sugar, 200 g
millet wine, 1000 ml

**Process**  Cut ginger into pieces. Soak the pieces along with sugar in millet wine and seal the container, put it in a cool, dry place for 7 days. Shake the container once daily during soaking. Filter the tincture and store it up for future administration.

**Directions**  Take 15 ml twice daily.

**Indications**  Hypofunction of stomach manifested by vomiting, anorexia, mild cold, and dysmenorrhea.

## Section 10 Hiccup

Hiccup refers to abrupt involuntary lowering of the diaphragm and closure of the sound-producing folds at the upper end of the trachea, producing a characteristic sound as the breath is drawn in. It is usually occur repeatedly, and may be caused by indigestion or more serious disorders. Hiccup is mostly due to adverse rising of stomach qi caused by either the injury or blockage of the stomach yang due to constitutional deficiency or overeating of raw and cold food. Sudden excessive eating of greasy or spicy food may also cause impairment of qi mechanism affecting the diaphragm because such a diet results in qi obstruction and retention of dryness and heat in middle jiao. Emotional disturbance with liver qi stagnation can cause an impaired qi mechanism because the stagnant liver qi attacks the stomach and causes the derangement of stomach qi. The deficiency of spleen yang and kidney yang with a decline of stomach accounts for another factor of hiccup because in such a case the clear qi can not normally ascend while the turbid qi is not lowers.

**Recipe** 1
**Ingredients**
spirit, 10 ml
**Directions**  Take 10 ml of spirit when hiccup occurs.
**Indication**  Hiccup due to cold evil.

**Recipe** 2
**Ingredients**
lemon, 1
spirit
**Process**  Soak lemon in right amount of spirit for a while. Then filter the tincture for future administration.
**Directions**  Remove the peel of the lemon and take it when suffering from hiccup.
**Indication**  Hiccup.

**Recipe** 3
**Ingredients**
Calyx Kaki, 9 g
millet wine
**Process**  Decoct persimmon calyxes with right amount of water.
**Directions**  Take the decoction with warm millet wine.
**Indication**  Hiccup.

**Recipe** 4
**Ingredients**
Sulphur, 5 g
Folium Artemisiae Argyi, 10 g
Rhizoma Zingiberis, 3 g
spirit

**Process**  Decoct sulphur and argyi leaves in right amount of spirit to get medicinal steam.

**Directions**  Have ginger slices in the mouth and inhale the steam. Once daily. One course consisting of three days.

**Indication**  Hiccup due to cold retention in the chest and diaphragm.

**Recipe** 5
**Ingredients**
Realgar, 10 g
spirit, 50 ml

**Process**  Grind realgar into powder. Decoct the powder in spirit to get medicinal steam.
**Directions**  Inhale the steam when hiccup occurs.
**Indication**  Hiccup.

## Section 11 Epigastric Pain

Epigastric pain, or gastric pain, refers to a syndrome manifested by frequent pain over the epigastric region. It is commonly seen in acute and chronic gastritis, gastric or duodenal ulcer, gastroneurosis and gastric cancer in modern medicine. Epigastric pain is mainly caused by the subsequent factors. Melancholy or emotional disturbance may cause the stagnation of liver qi and dysfunction of the liver to maintain the free flow of qi, leading to incoordination between stomach qi and liver qi which results in poor descending of stomach qi. Improper intake of cold or raw food or intake of unclean food may impair the spleen and stomach, resulting in poor transportation and transformation by the spleen and food retention in the middle jiao. Constitutional deficiency of the spleen and stomach in combination with cold invasion may give rise to accumulation of cold in the stomach and failure of the stomach qi to descend, thus causing pain in the epigastrium.

**Recipe** 1
**Ingredients**
Herba Taraxaci, 25 g
millet wine

**Process**  Decoct dandelion herb with water.
**Directions**  Take one recipe along with 5 ml of millet wine, daily. 7 days consisted of one

course.

**Indications**  Epigastric pain, vomiting, regurgitation due to gastric ulcer.

**Recipe** 2
**Ingredients**
Zaocys, 1
rice wine
**Process**  Soak black-tail snake in spirit and seal the container, put it in a cool, dry place for over one year.
**Directions**  Take 10 ml twice daily.
**Indication**  Gastrospasm.

**Recipe** 3
**Ingredients**
Pericarpium Zanthoxyli, 30 g
millet wine, 500 ml
**Process**  Cook bunge pricklyash peel, soak it in millet wine, put it in a cool, dry place for 7 days. Shake the container once daily during soaking. Filter the tincture and store it up for future administration.
**Directions**  Take 10 ml twice daily.
**Indication**  Cold pain in the epigastric region.

**Recipe** 4
**Ingredients**
Rhizoma Zingiberis, 30 g
Radix Glycyrrhizae, 30 g
Radix et Rhizoma Rhei, 30 g
Radix Ginseng, 20 g
Radix Aconiti Praeparata, 20 g
millet wine, 1000 ml
**Process**  Grind the above ingredients except millet wine into fine powder. Soak the powder in millet wine and seal the container, put it in a cool, dry place for 5 days. Shake the container once daily during soaking. Filter the tincture and store it up for future administration.
**Directions**  Take 10 ml twice daily.
**Indications**  Cold pain in the epigastric region, constipation, chronic dysentery.

**Recipe** 5
**Ingredients**
Rhizoma Pinelliae, 30 g
Radix Scutellariae, 30 g

Rhizoma Zingiberis, 20 g

Radix Ginseng, 20 g

Rhizoma Coptidis, 6 g

Fructus Jujubae, 10 g

spirits, 1000 ml

**Process**  Pound the above ingredients into pieces, fill them in a gauze bag. Soak the bag in spirit and seal the container, put it in a cool, dry place for 5 days. Shake the container once daily during soaking. Filter the tincture and add 500 ml of water, store it up for future administration.

**Directions**  Take 20 ml twice daily.

**Indications**  Epigastric pain, distention of the epigastric region, regurgitation, nausea, vomiting, borborygmus, anorexia, lassitude and fatigue.

### Recipe 6

**Ingredients**

Fructus Foenicuii, 100 g

Rhizoma Acori Graminei, 100 g

Fructus Aurantii, 100 g

spirit, 1000 ml

**Process**  Soak citron fruit, common fennel fruit and grassleaved sweetflag rhizome in spirit and seal the container, put it in a cool, dry place for 10 days. Shake the container once daily during soaking. Filter the tincture and store it up for future administration.

**Directions**  Take 10 ml after meals daily.

**Indications**  Chronic gastritis, gastroptosis manifested by distention and fullness sensation in the epigastric region.

### Recipe 7

**Ingredients**

Rhizoma Alpiniae Officinarum, 12 g

Rhizoma Chuanxiong, 12 g

spirit, 500 ml

**Process**  Put galangal rhizome and szechuan lovage rhizome along with spirit in a container. Steam the container in boiling water for 30 minutes.

**Directions**  Take 5 to 10 ml before meals daily.

**Indication**  Recurrent stomachache.

### Recipe 8

**Ingredients**

Fructus Foenicuii, 50 g

spirits, 500 ml

**Process**  Soak common fennel fruit in spirit and seal the container, put it in a cool, dry place for

7 days. Shake the container once daily during soaking. Filter the tincture and store it up for future administration.

**Directions**   Take right amount of tincture once daily.
**Indication**   Epigastric pain.

### Recipe 9
**Ingredients**
Semen Nelumbinis, 250 g
lard, 6 g
rice wine, 6 g
**Process**   Mix lotus seed along with lard and rice wine in a container. Cook them in boiling water until they are done.
**Directions**   Take the seed daily. One course consisting of one month.
**Indications**   Gastric ulcer or gastric hemorrhage (restoration stage).

### Recipe 10
**Ingredients**
sugarcane juice, 10 ml
grape wine, 10 ml
**Process**   Mix sugarcane and grape wine equally.
**Directions**   Take the mixture twice daily.
**Indication**   Chronic gastritis.

### Recipe 11
**Ingredients**
egg, 12
crystal sugar, 500 g
millet wine, 500 ml
**Process**   Remove the eggshells and mix with sugar and wine equally. Cook the mixture until it becomes brown.
**Directions**   Take one spoon before meals daily.
**Indication**   Gastrospasm.

### Recipe 12
**Ingredients**
Semen Gossypii, 20 g
spirit, 5 ml
**Process**   Put cotton seed in a container. Add 60 ml of water in. Decoct the mixture until 20 ml of decoction left. Mix the decoction and spirit equally.
**Directions**   Take the decoction once daily.

**Indication**  Epigastric pain.

**Recipe** 13
**Ingredients**
common carp, 1
crystal sugar, 50 g
spirit

**Process**  Remove the internal organs of the carp, cut it into slices. Soak them in warm spirit and seal the container, put it in a cool, dry place for several hours. Filter the tincture and add crystal sugar in it, stir the mixture equally and store it up for future administration.

**Directions**  Take 10 ml 2 hours after meals, three times daily.
**Indication**  Chronic gastroduodenal ulcer.

**Recipe** 14
**Ingredients**
pork corp

**Process**  Remove the meat and pound the bones into pieces. Parch the bones with their nature retained. Grind the parched bones into fine powder for later use.
**Directions**  Take 10 to 15 g with 30 ml of millet wine twice daily.
**Indication**  Gastroduodenal ulcer.

**Recipe** 15
**Ingredients**
Pericarpium Juglandis, 60 g
spirit, 250 ml

**Process**  Soak green peel of walnut kernel in 250 ml of spirit and seal the container, put it in a cool, dry place for 7 days. Shake the container once daily during soaking. Filter the tincture and store it up for future administration.
**Directions**  Take 3 ml once daily.
**Indication**  Epigastric pain.

**Recipe** 16
**Ingredients**
Herba Coriandri, 1000 g
grape wine, 500 ml

**Process**  Soak coriander in grape wine and seal the container, put it in a cool, dry place for 3 days. Shake the container once daily during soaking. Filter the tincture and store it up for future administration.
**Directions**  Take 15 ml in case of stomachache.

**Indication** Epigastric pain.

**Recipe** 17
**Ingredients**
litchi, 5
spirit, 50 ml
**Process** Remove the peel of the fruit and soak them in 100 ml of water in a container with the lid covered. Decoct them over a slow fire until it has been brought to several times of boils.
**Directions** Take the fruit warmly.
**Indication** Epigastric pain, gastroptosis.

## Section 12 Abdominal Pain

Abdominal pain refers to the pain involving the area below the epigastrium and above the suprapubic hair margin. Clinically, it is very commonly encountered in various diseases. It can be seen in both acute and chronic enteritis, gastrointestinal spasm, intestinal neurosis and indigestion in terms of modern medicine. It is mostly caused by overeating of cold or raw food, or invasion of exogenous pathogenic cold into the abdomen. The constraining and stagnant property of cold causes the obstruction of qi mechanism which gives rise to pain. Overeating of greasy oily food or unclean food can cause food retention which will turn into heat retained in the intestine. The intestinal heat blocks the normal circulation of intestinal qi and leads to the onset of abdominal pain. Constitutional yang deficiency and spleen yang deficiency in particular can also cause abdominal pain because of the dysfunction of both spleen and stomach.

**Recipe** 1
**Ingredients**
mussel
Herba Allii Tuberosi
millet wine
**Process** Soak mussel in right amount of millet wine. Decoct mussel along with Chinese chives until they are done.
**Directions** Take the above medicinal diet once daily.
**Indication** Cold pain in the lower abdomen in women.

**Recipe** 2
**Ingredients**
Rhizoma Cyperi, 30 g
spirit, 500 ml

**Process**  Soak nutgrass flatsedge rhizome in spirit and seal the container, put it in a cool, dry place for 7 days. Shake the container once daily during soaking. Filter the tincture and store it up for future administration.

**Directions**  Take 20 ml three times daily.

**Indication**  Pain in the lower abdomen.

### Recipe 3
**Ingredients**

Fructus Chaenomelis, 120 g

Fructus Foenicuii, 90 g

Pericarpium Citri Reticulatae Viride, 60 g

millet wine

**Process**  Grind chaenomeles fruit, common fennel fruit and green tangerine orange peel into fine powder. Mix it with Mel to make pills the size of soya beans.

**Directions**  Take 3 pills along with warm millet wine, twice daily.

**Indications**  Distending pain in the lower abdomen or pain in the abdomen and hypochondria.

### Recipe 4
**Ingredients**

Fructus Amomi, 30 g

spirit, 500 ml

**Process**  Pound amomum fruit into pieces. Soak them in spirits and seal the container, put it in a cool, dry place for 7 days. Shake the container once daily during soaking. Filter the tincture and store it up for future administration.

**Directions**  Take 10 ml after meals twice daily.

**Indication**  Distending pain in the epigastric region.

### Recipe 5
**Ingredients**

Fructus Tsaoko, 10 g

Pericarpium Citri Reticulatae, 5 g

Fructus Crataegi, 5 g

spirit, 250 ml

**Process**  Soak tsaoko cardamon, tangerine peel and hawthorn fruit in spirit and seal the container, put it in a cool, dry place for 7 days. Shake the container once daily during soaking. Filter the tincture and store it up for future administration.

**Directions**  Take 10 ml twice daily.

**Indication**  Distending pain in the epigastric region.

### Recipe 6
**Ingredients**
Fructus Mume, 30 g
millet wine, 100 ml
**Process**  Steam black plums along with millet wine for 20 minutes.
**Directions**  Take 10 ml of tincture warmly, twice daily.
**Indication**  Ascaris abdominal pain.

### Recipe 7
**Ingredients**
Fructus Mori, 200 g
spirit
**Process**  Grind dried mulberries into fine powder.
**Directions**  Take 10 g along with warm spirit to get mild sweat, once daily.
**Indication**  Abdominal pain due to cold retention.

### Recipe 8
**Ingredients**
Flos Caryophylli, 2 grains
millet wine, 50 ml
**Process**  Put cloves in millet wine in a container. Steam the container in boiling water for 10 minutes.
**Directions**  Take 10 ml of millet wine warmly.
**Indications**  Abdominal pain, distention of the abdomen, vomiting and diarrhea due to attacking of cold evil.

### Recipe 9
**Ingredients**
Fructus Anisi Stellati, 9 g
spirit
**Process**  Soak star anise fruit in small amount of spirit. Then decoct them with water.
**Directions**  Take the decoction once daily.
**Indication**  Abdominal pain due to attacking of cold evil.

### Recipe 10
**Ingredients**
Pericarpium Zanthoxyli, 9 grains
Fructus Jujubae, 20 g
millet wine
**Process**  Pound bunge pricklyash peel and jujubes into mash.

**Directions**　Take the mash along with warm millet wine, once daily.
**Indication**　Abdominal pain due to attacking of cold evil.

**Recipe** 11
**Ingredients**
Rhizoma Zingiberis, 20 g
Bulbus Allii, 10 g
spirit
**Process**　Pound ginger and green onion into mash.
**Directions**　Take the mash along with warm spirit.
**Indication**　Abdominal pain due to attacking of cold evil.

**Recipe** 12
**Ingredients**
Rhizoma Zingiberis, 10 g
brown sugar, 60 g
spirit
**Process**　Soak ginger in the syrup and add small amount of spirit.
**Directions**　Take the mixture warmly, once daily.
**Indications**　Cold pain in the abdomen, cold limbs, diarrhea.

**Recipe** 13
**Ingredients**
Pericarpium Zanthoxyli, 30 g
Semen Phaseoli Radiati, 30 g
millet wine
**Process**　Grind bunge pricklyash peel and mung beans into fine powder.
**Directions**　Take 3 g of the powder along with warm millet wine (right amount), twice daily.
**Indication**　Abdominal pain due to attacking of cold evil.

**Recipe** 14
**Ingredients**
Arillus Longan, 100 g
rice wine
**Process**　Parch longan aril with its nature retained. Grind the parched fruit into fine powder.
**Directions**　Take 10 g of the powder along with warm rice wine.
**Indication**　Abdominal pain due to attacking of cold evil.

**Recipe** 15
**Ingredients**

Rhizoma Zingiberis, 50 g

grape wine, 500 g

**Process**  Pound ginger into mash. Soak the mash in wine and seal the container, put it in a cool, dry place for 3 days. Shake the container once daily during soaking. Filter the tincture and store it up for future administration.

**Directions**  Take 50 ml once daily.

**Indications**  Abdominal pain due to attacking of cold evil, belching, hiccup.

**Recipe 16**

**Ingredients**

Fructus Citri Sarcodactylis, 300 g

spirit, 1000 ml

**Process**  Wash finger citron clean and cut into slices. Soak the dried citron in spirit and seal the container, put it in a cool, dry place for 15 days. Shake the container once every three days. Then remove the dregs and store the extracts up for later use.

**Directions**  Take 15 ml twice daily.

**Indications**  Incoordination between liver and stomach manifested by distending pain in the abdomen, chest and hypochondria.

**Recipe 17**

**Ingredients**

Flos Caryophylli, 2 grains

Fructus Crataegi, 6 g

millet wine, 50 ml

**Process**  Put the above ingredients in a container. Steam it for 10 minutes. Remove the dregs for later use.

**Directions**  Take the tincture warmly.

**Indications**  Abdominal pain, distention of the abdomen, vomiting and diarrhea due to cold evil.

**Recipe 18**

**Ingredients**

red bayberry

spirit

**Process**  Soak red bayberries in a right amount of spirits.

**Directions**  Take 2 to 3 bayberries and drink 10 ml of the tincture once daily. One course consisting of 7 days.

**Indication**  Abdominal pain due to attacking of cold evil.

**Recipe** 19
**Ingredients**
Bulbus Allii, 1500 g
vinegar, 300 ml
spirit, 300 ml

**Process**  Mix vinegar and spirit equally in a container. Put garlic in and seal the container for 10 days.

**Directions**  Take 3 to 5 garlic in case of abdominal pain.

**Indication**  Abdominal pain due to attacking of cold evil.

## Section 13 Pain in the Chest and Hypochondria

This section embraces precordial pain, distention in the chest and hypochondriac pain. The first two symptoms are partly described in section 18. Hypochondriac pain refers to a painful sensation either on one side or both sides of the hypochondrium. It is included in hepatopathy, biliary disorders, intercostal neuralgia, etc. in modern medicine. The onset of hypochondriac pain is mostly due to melancholy or violent anger that leads to the failure of the liver to spread qi freely, thus resulting in qi stagnation. Invasion of exogenous pathogenic damp-heat, improper diet such as overeating or excessive alcoholic indulgence may cause accumulation of damp-heat in the liver and gallbladder and misachieved free flow of qi. Abrupt stumbling or twisting may give rise to impairment of channels and collaterals in the hypochondriac region, resulting in stagnation of qi and blood and obstruction of channels and collaterals. However, prolonged illness with poor constitution, overstrain and insufficiency of both qi and blood can also be the cause of the poor nourishment of the liver.

**Recipe** 1
**Ingredients**
Herba Allii Tuberosi, 20 g
spirits, 5 ml

**Process**  Extract the Chinese chives into mash to get juice.

**Directions**  Take the juice with spirits warmly, once daily.

**Indication**  Precordial pain.

**Recipe** 2
**Ingredients**
Semen Litchi, 1

spirits, right amount

**Process**  Parch the litchi seed with its nature retained. Grind the parched pit into fine powder.

**Directions**  Take the powder with warm spirits.

**Indication**  Precordial pain.

### Recipe 3
**Ingredients**
Concha Cipangopaludina Chinensis, 10
spirits, right amount

**Process**  Wash the shells of snails clean. Parch the shells with their nature retained. Grind the parched shells into fine powder.

**Directions**  Take 3 g of the powder with spirits.

**Indication**  Precordial pain due to retention of damp and phlegm.

### Recipe 4
**Ingredients**
Pericarpium Zanthoxyli, 20 g
Semen Phaseoli Radiati, 20 g
millet wine, right amount

**Process**  Grind the dried bunge pricklyash peel and mung bean into fine powder.

**Directions**  Take 5 g of the powder with right a mount of millet wine twice daily.

**Indications**  Precordial pain and cold pain in the epigastric region.

### Recipe 5
**Ingredients**
Massa Fermentata Medicinalis
Rhizoma Cyperi
Resina Olibani
spirits

**Process**  Grind a right amount of medicated leaven, nutgrass flatsedge rhizome and olibanum into fine powder.

**Directions**  Take a right amount of the powder with warm spirits.

**Indications**  Precordial pain and pain in the epigastric region.

### Recipe 6
**Ingredients**
Fructus Mume, 3
Pericarpium Zanthoxyli, 7 grains
millet wine, right amount

**Process**  Pound black plums and /bunge pricklyash peel into mash.

**Directions**  Take the mash with warm millet wine.
**Indication**  Chronic epigastric pain.

### Recipe 7
**Ingredients**

Radix Aucklandiae, 10 g

Radix Curcumae, 10 g

millet wine, right amount

**Process**  Make decoction with curcuma root and costus root with water.
**Directions**  Take the decoction with warm millet wine.
**Indication**  Distending pain in the chest.

### Recipe 8
**Ingredients**

Radix Ziziphi Spinosae, 30 g

Rhizoma Pinelliae, 10 g

millet wine, right amount

**Process**  Decoct spine date root and pinellia tuber with water.
**Directions**  Take the decoction with warm millet wine, twice daily.
**Indications**  Chest pain accompanied by palpitation.

### Recipe 9
**Ingredients**

Retinervus Citri Reticulatae Fructus, 3 g

Radix Angelicae Sinensis, 3 g

Flos Carthami, 3 g

millet wine, right amount

**Process**  Grind tangerine pith, safflower and Chinese angelica into powder.
**Directions**  Take the powder with warm millet wine, twice daily.
**Indications**  Chest distress, pain in the hypochondria, intercostal neuralgia.

### Recipe 10
**Ingredients**

Pericarpium Zanthoxyli, 7 grains

Fructus Jujubae, 3

Semen Armeniacae Amarum, 7

millet wine, right amount

**Process**  Pound bunge pricklyash peel, jujubes and bitter apricot seed into mash.
**Directions**  Take the mash with warm millet wine.
**Indications**  Distending pain in the chest and abdomen.

**Recipe** 11
**Ingredients**
Fructus Luffae, 100 g
spirits, right amount
**Process**　Parch the towel gourds with their nature retained. Grind the parched gourds into fine powder.
**Directions**　Take 10 g of the powder with warm spirits.
**Indications**　Pain in the chest and hypochondria.

Recipe 12
**Ingredients**
Fructus Foenicuii, 60 g
Fructus Aurantii Immaturus, 15 g
millet wine, right amount
**Process**　Grind the immature bitter oranges and common fennel fruit into fine powder and then mix the powder equally.
**Directions**　Take 6 g of the powder with warm millet wine.
**Indication**　Pain in the hypochondria.

Recipe 13
**Ingredients**
Fructus Kochiae, 6 g
millet wine, right amount
**Process**　Grind broom cypress fruit into fine powder.
**Directions**　Take the powder with warm millet wine.
**Indication**　Pain in the hypochondria.

Recipe 14
**Ingredients**
Excrementa Bombycum, 100 g
millet wine, 500 ml
**Process**　Bake silkworm excrement over a slow fire. Fill the dried silkworm excrement in a gauze bag, and then soak it in 500 ml of millet wine and seal the container, put it in a cool, dry place for 7 to 10 days. Shake the container once daily during soaking. Filter the tincture and store it up for future administration.
**Directions**　Take right amount of the tincture twice daily.
**Indication**　Neuralgia and rheumatalgia, numbness of the extremities.

**Recipe** 15
**Ingredients**
Fructus Mori, 500 g
Ramulus Mori, 1000 g
brown sugar, 250 g
spirit, 1000 ml

**Process**  Cut mulberry twigs into short branches. Fill mulberry and mulberry twigs in a bottle. Add brown sugar along with spirit in and seal the bottle for one month. Shake the bottle every three days.

**Directions**  Take 10 ml of the tincture twice daily. One course consists of two months.

**Indication**  Neuroarthropathy.

**Recipe** 16
**Ingredients**
Semen Canavaliae, 15 g
millet wine

**Process**  Parch sword beans with their nature retained and grind them into powder.

**Directions**  Take 3 g along with millet wine three times daily.

**Indication**  Intercostal neuralgia.

## Section 14 Diarrhea

Diarrhea refers to frequent bowel evacuation or the passage of abnormally soft or liquid feces. There are two types: acute and chronic in the clinic. Diarrhea of abrupt onset occurring in otherwise healthy persons is most often related to an infectious process. A variety of accompanying symptoms include fever, headache, anorexia, vomiting, malaise, and myalgia. Acute diarrhea presumed to be of viral etiology typically persists for a period of one to three days and death is extremely rare. Bacterial diarrhea may be suspected if there is a history of a similar and simultaneous illness in individuals who have shared contaminated food with the patient. Protozoal infections may also be responsible for acute diarrhea. Ulcerative colitis and regional enteritis may begin as acute diarrhea. Diarrhea may be caused by a variety of drugs. Diarrhea due to diverticulitis is usually accompanied by fever, tenesmus, and rectal urgency, together with cramps and tenderness in the left lower quadrant. When there is no evidence of acute inflammation, diarrhea in the presence of colonic diverticula is probably due to a spastic colon. In elderly and debilitated individuals with fecal impaction, the presenting symptom may be the frequent expulsion of small amounts of liquid stool overflowing from colonic distention behind the impaction. Fecal incontinence due to anal sphincter impairment is a problem that may be encountered in certain neurologic disorders or local surgical procedures. Acute psychological stress can cause diarrhea at any age. Diarrhea persisting for weeks or months, whether constant or intermittent, may be a functional symptom or a manifestation of serious illness. Abdominal tenderness and fever suggest the presence of inflammation. When there is involvement of the large bowel, the major diseases to be considered comprise ulcerative colitis, Crohn's disease of the small intestine may involve one or more of its segments. Other diarrheal conditions which may resemble Crohn's disease radiographically include tuberculous and fungal enteritis, lymphosarcoma, amyloidosis, and argentaffin tumors of the small bowel. prolonged diarrhea without evidence of inflammation may reflect impairment of absorption, secretion, or digestion. Endocrine disorders that may be accompanied by chronic diarrhea include thyrotoxicosis, diabetes mellitus, adrenal insufficiency, and hypoparathyroidism. Habitual cathartic abuse must be suspected when the cause of prolonged diarrhea remains perplexing.

According to traditional Chinese medicine, the condition is mainly caused by dysfunctions of the spleen and stomach. Acute diarrhea is mostly due to an improper diet related to intake of cold raw food or unclean food, or due to invasion of pathogenic cold, dampness and summer heat, especially dampness. These factors can cause obstruction of the spleen yang impair the function of the spleen and stomach, leading to poor function of the spleen in transformation and transportation and nonseparation of the turbid from the clean in the intestine to form diarrhea. Chronic diarrhea is mostly due to impairment of the spleen by over worry or constitutional deficiency of the spleen and stomach. Nevertheless, the dysfunction of liver in maintaining free flow of qi, and stagnant liver qi attacking the stomach can lead to its overacting on the spleen and stomach. Yang deficiency of the kidney after prolonged illness causes inadequate warming on the spleen and stomach to do digestion. Therefore, diarrhea is the consequence of dysfunction of the spleen and stomach.

**Recipe** 1
**Ingredients**
brown sugar, right amount
spirit, right amount
**Process** Dissolve the brown sugar in spirit.
**Directions** Take the solution when it is warm, twice daily.
**Indication** Diarrhea of cold type manifested by watery stools.

**Recipe** 2
**Ingredients**
dried persimmon, 2
spirit, right amount
**Process** Steam the persimmons when they are done.
**Directions** Take the persimmons along with right amount of spirit twice daily.
**Indication** Diarrhea of cold type revealed by watery stools.

**Recipe** 3
**Ingredients**

Flos Caryophylli, 2 grains

millet wine, 50 ml

**Process**  Soak cloves in millet wine in an earthen jar, cover the lid and then steam it for 10 minutes. After it cools, filter the decoction and store it up for future administration.

**Directions**  Take 50 ml of the millet wine warmly, twice daily.

**Indications**  Diarrhea due to suffering from cold marked by diarrhea and vomiting, distending pain in the abdomen.

### Recipe 4
**Ingredients**

red bayberry, right amount

spirit, right amount

**Process**  Soak the bayberries in spirit and seal the container, put it in a cool, dry place for 7 days. Shake the container once daily during soaking. Filter the tincture and store it up for future administration.

**Directions**  Take one or two red bayberries twice daily.

**Indication**  Diarrhea.

### Recipe 5
**Ingredients**

egg, 1

sugar, 10 g

spirit, 100 ml

**Process**  Remove the shell of the egg and mix it with sugar and spirit equally. light the mixture until it is done.

**Directions**  Take the egg once daily.

**Indication**  Diarrhea.

### Recipe 6
**Ingredients**

Rhizoma Zingiberis, 3 g

brown sugar, 50 g

millet wine, 250 ml

vinegar, right amount

**Process**  Decoct the ingredients until they are done.

**Directions**  Take 20 ml of the decoction warmly, twice daily.

**Indication**  Chronic diarrhea.

### Recipe 7
**Ingredients**

Rhizoma Zingiberis, 120 g

rice wine, 30 g

**Process**  Wash the fresh ginger clean and cut into slices. Soak the slices in rice wine for 5 minutes and then rub the patient's extremities with ginger slices until the skin becomes congested.

**Directions**  Apply rubbing method twice or three times daily. One course consisting of 3 to 5 days.

**Indication**  Diarrhea due to acute gastroenteritis.

Recipe 8

**Ingredients**

argyi wool

spirit

**Process**  Pound right amount of argyi wool the size of a small cake. Soak the argyi wool in spirit for one hour.

**Directions**  Apply argyi wool cakes on Shenque(RN8) and Zhongwan(RN12) and then heat the points with moxa sticks.

**Indication**  Diarrhea.

Recipe 9

**Ingredients**

rosin, 6 g

spirit

**Process**  Grind rosin into fine powder. Mix it with right amount of spirit.

**Directions**  Apply the mixture on Shenque(RN8) once daily.

**Indication**  Diarrhea.

Recipe 10

**Ingredients**

Folium Artemisiae Argyi, right amount

spirit

**Process**  Wash argyi leaves clean and pound into mash. Put it in a pot and add right amount of spirit. Cook the mash until it is hot. Fill it in a gauze bag and apply the bag on Shenque(RN8) when it is warm.

**Directions**  Heat the point for continuous 15 minutes twice or three times daily. One course consisting of 3 to 5 days.

**Indication**  Diarrhea due to acute gastroenteritis.

Recipe 11

**Ingredients**

Bulbus Allii, right amount

spirit

**Process**  Wash green onion clean and pound into mash. Put it in a pot and add right amount of spirit. Cook the mash until it is hot. Fill it in a gauze bag and apply the bag on Shenque(RN8) when it is warm.

**Directions**  Heat the point for continuous 15 minutes twice or three times daily. One course consisting of 3 to 5 days.

**Indication**  Diarrhea due to acute gastroenteritis.

## Section 15 Jaundice

Jaundice or icterus, refers to the yellow pigmentation of the skin or scleras by bilirubin. This in turn is a result of elevated levels of bilirubin in the bloodstream. Jaundice may be brought to clinical attention by a darkening of the urine or a yellow discoloration of the skin or sclera; the latter often is the site where clinical icterus may first be detected. Jaundice is mostly seen in the infantile, the young and the middle aged. It may result from exogenous as well as endogenous pathogenic factors. Accumulation of exogenous pathogenic damp-heat in the liver and gallbladder with dampness retention and heat steaming impairs the liver in maintaining the free flow of qi so the bile floods to cause jaundice. This is known as yang type of jaundice. Impairment of the spleen and stomach and dysfunction of the spleen in transformation and transportation due to overstrain, over thinking or improper diet lead to dampness retention and qi stagnation in the liver and gallbladder resulting in the unsmooth flow and excretion of bile that floods also to the superficies of the body to develop into jaundice. This known as the yin type of jaundice.

### Recipe 1
**Ingredients**
Herba Lophatheri, 30 g
spirit, 500 ml

**Process**  Wash lophatherum clean and cut into lengths of 2 cm long. Soak them in 500 ml of spirit and seal the container, put it in a cool, dry place for 3 days. Shake the container once daily during soaking. Filter the tincture and store it up for future administration.

**Directions**  Take 10 ml twice daily.

**Indication**  Dark urine and jaundice.

### Recipe 2
**Ingredients**
Cipangopaludina Chinensis, 10-20
millet wine, 15 ml

**Process**   Wash the snails clean and take their meat. Mix the meat with millet wine and cook over a slow fire until it is done.

**Directions**   Take the meat and soup once daily.

**Indication**   Jaundice of damp-heat type.

**Recipe** 3

**Ingredients**

crab claw

spirit

**Process**   Parch the crab claws with their nature retained. Grind the parched claws into fine powder and mix with spirit to make pills the size of a Chinese parasol fruit.

**Directions**   Take 50 pills with water twice daily.

**Indication**   Jaundice of damp-heat type.

## Section 16 Spontaneous Perspiration and Night Sweat

Spontaneous perspiration and night sweat are considered in the term of sweat syndrome in traditional Chinese medicine. It is a condition of poor opening and closing of skin pores with heavy perspiration due to the imbalance of yin and yang of the body, and the disharmony between the nutritive and defensive systems. Spontaneous perspiration is characterized by perspiration that can be worsened by exertion, while the latter characterized by perspiration during sleep at night that stops by itself when the patient is wakened. Spontaneous perspiration and night sweat may be seen in hyperthyroidism, vegetative nerve dysfunction, hypoglycemia, tuberculosis, rheumatic fever as well and at the acute and rehabilitative stages of some infectious diseases. There are many factors which may lead to sweat syndrome. Poor defensive yang energy and disharmony between the nutritive and defensive systems due to constitutional yang deficiency with poor function of skin pores in opening and closing and invasion of exogenous pathogenic wind; turbid dampness retention in the middle jiao turning into heat to steam the superficial portion of the body due to impairment and dysfunction of the spleen and stomach in transforming and transporting caused by either improper food intake or invasion of exogenous pathogenic dampness; or dormant heat in the interior with unrecovered yin qi of the body due to severe or lingering illness, may cause the sweat syndrome. Moreover, over consumption of kidney essence due to excessive sexual indulgence or heat retention in the interior of the body due to the use of drugs that have heat property can also cause over consumption of yin blood. Therefore, sweating appears when yin does not match the hyperactive yang in the body.

**Recipe** 1

**Ingredients**

Misgurnus Anguillicaudatus, 250 g

rice wine

**Process** Wash the loaches clean and decoct them with right amount of rice wine.
**Directions** Take the loaches once daily.
**Indication** Night sweat.

### Recipe 2
**Ingredients**
Radix Ginseng, 30 g
spirit, 500 ml

**Process** Fill a gauze bag with ginseng and cook it with spirit in a container. Then seal the container for 7 days.
**Directions** Take 5 ml twice daily.
**Indications** Deficiency of spleen qi marked by spontaneous perspiration, aversion to cold, dyspnea due to activities, general weakness, sallow face.

### Recipe 3
**Ingredients**
pork, 250 g
rice wine, 500 ml
white sugar
salt

**Process** Cook the pork with rice wine until it is done. Mix right amount of white sugar and salt to make it delicious.
**Directions** Take the pork once daily. One course consisting of two days.
**Indication** Night sweat.

### Recipe 4
**Ingredients**
Semen Sojae Preparatum, 250 g
rice wine, 1000 ml

**Process** Stir-fry the fermented soya beans and then Soak them in rice wine and seal the container, put it in a cool, dry place for 3 days. Shake the container once daily during soaking. Filter the tincture and store it up for future administration.
**Directions** Take 10 ml of the rice wine twice daily.
**Indication** Night sweat.

### Recipe 5
**Ingredients**
soft-shelled turtle, 1
millet wine

**Process**  Kill the turtle to get blood.
**Directions**  Take the blood with right amount of warm millet wine once daily.
**Indication**  Night sweat.

## Section 17 Constipation

Constipation refers to a condition in which bowel evacuation occur infrequently, or in which the feces are hard and small, or where passage of feces causes difficulty or pain. A review of the patient's habits often reveals contributory and correctable causes, such as insufficient dietary roughage, lack of exercise, suppression of defecatory urges arising at inconvenient moments, inadequate allotment of time for full defecation, and prolonged travel. When the patient also has symptoms such as fatigue, malaise, headaches, or anorexia, the possibility should be considered that such symptoms reflect an underlying depression of which constipation is but one component. Decreased colonic motility is responsible for the constipation associated with the use of parasympatholytic drugs, spinal cord injury, scleroderma, and Hirschsprung's disease. Hemorrhoids, anal fissures, perineal abscesses, and rectal strictures often prevent easy and adequate stool evacuation. When constipation and tenesmus of recent onset are reported, the possibility of carcinoma of the rectum or descending colon must be seriously considered. Other mechanical causes of constipation include volvulus of the sigmoid colon, diverticultis, intussusception, and hernias. A variety of metabolic abnormalities, such as hypothyroidism, hypercalcemia, hypokalemia, porphyria lead poisoning, and dehydration are often associated with constipation. Tremendous fecal retention and impaction may occur in certain neurologic disorders.

Constitutional excess of yang, alcoholic indulgence, habitual intake of greasy spicy food or remnant heat after febrile disease may all cause heat accumulation in the stomach and intestine and consumption of the body fluid, leading the dryness of intestines as well as dry stools. Either emotional disturbance such as anxiety and depression, or lack of physical exertion may cause stagnation of qi impairing the function of the large intestine in transmitting. As a result, the wastes are retained inside and unable to move downward, causing the constipation. Deficiency of qi and blood resulted from illness or delivery causes two subsequent conditions of deficiency. Specifically, qi deficiency leads to weakness of the large intestine in transmission, while blood deficiency weakens the moistening of the large intestine in descending wastes. Deficiency of yang qi in the aged causes accumulation of interior cold. The stagnant cold can not help the transformation and distribution of qi, resulting in constipation.

**Recipe** 1
**Ingredients**
Pericarpium Citri Reticulatae, right amount
spirit
**Process**  Soak the tangerine peel in spirit and then decoct it until the peel becomes pliable. Bake

the peel and then grind the dried peel into fine powder.

**Directions**  Take 10 g of the powder with right amount of warm spirit once daily.

**Indication**  Constipation.

### Recipe 2
**Ingredients**

Radix et Rhizoma Rhei, 50 g

Semen Sojae Preparatum, 500 g

spirit, 1500 ml

**Process**  Grind the rhubarb into fine powder. Fill a gauze bag with fermented soya beans and rhubarb powder with the mouth of the bag fastened, then soak it in spirit and seal the container for 21 days.

**Directions**  Take 5 ml twice daily. One course consisting of 5 days.

**Indication**  Constipation due to sthenic heat in gastrointestinal tract. Contraindicated to cases such as pregnant women.

### Recipe 3
**Ingredients**

pine nut, right amount

old wine, 5 ml

**Process**  Pound the pine nuts into mash and then mix it with old wine.

**Directions**  Take the mixture twice daily.

**Indication**  Constipation.

### Recipe 4
**Ingredients**

Semen Persicae, 60 g

rice wine, 100 g

**Process**  Pound the peach kernels into mash and then soak it rice wine and seal the container for 10 days.

**Directions**  Take 20 ml twice daily.

**Indication**  Constipation due to postpartum deficiency of blood.

### Recipe 5
**Ingredients**

Fructus Cannabis, 500 g

rice wine, 1000 g

**Process**  Grind hemp seed into powder and soak it in rice wine for 7 days.

**Directions**  Take 20 ml twice daily.

**Indication**  Constipation due to senile or postpartum deficiency of blood.

**Recipe 6**
**Ingredients**
young bamboo, 120 g
spirit, 1000 g
**Process** Cut young bamboo into pieces. Soak them in spirit and seal the container for 12 days. Shake the container once every six days.
**Directions** Take 20 ml twice daily.
**Indications** Constipation, primary hypertension, hemorrhoid.

**Recipe 7**
**Ingredients**
pine nut, 70 g
millet wine, 500 g
**Process** Stir-fry the pine nuts and then pound into mash. Mix the mash with millet wine and decoct over a slow fire until it slightly boils. After it cools, seal the mouth of the container for 3 days. Remove the dregs and store the tincture for later use.
**Directions** Take 20 to 30 ml with water three times daily.
**Indications** Constipation, weakness, thirst, dizziness, cough with little sputum, xerosis cutis, palpitation, night sweat.

**Recipe 8**
**Ingredients**
Fructus Lycii, 750 g
Fructus Cannabis, 750 g
Radix Rehmanniae, 450 g
spirit, 4000 ml
**Process** Cut wolfberry fruit, hemp seed and rehmanniae root into pieces and steam them until they are done. After the pieces cool, soak them in spirit and seal the container for 7 days.
**Directions** Take 10 ml once daily.
**Indication** Constipation, general weakness, sallow face, lassitude and fatigue, dizziness, dry mouth, anorexia.

**Recipe 9**
**Ingredients**
Radix Rehmanniae
Rhizoma Zingiberis
suet, 150 g
Mel, 75 g
rice wine, 1000 ml

**Process**  Extract rehmannia root and ginger to get 70 g of juice each. Put rice wine in an earthenware pot over a slow fire and add suet in at the same time. Then mix with the juice of rehmannia root and ginger equally. Bring it to several boils. Cook the honey until it is done. Add honey in the mixture and mix it equally. Seal the container for 3 days.

**Directions**  Take 20 to 30 ml three times daily.

**Indications**  Constipation, anorexia, restlessness and thirst, cough with dryness sensation in the throat, weight loss.

**Recipe** 10

**Ingredients**

Semen Armeniacae Amarum, 60 g

Mel, 60 g

Radix Rehmanniae

Fructus Jujubae, 30 g

Rhizoma Zingiberis

peanut oil, 40 g

spirit, 1500 ml

**Process**  Cut fresh rehmannia root and ginger and extract their juice, 150 g and 40 g respectively. Pound jujubes and sweet apricot seed into mash. Put the juice of ginger in a china jar, mix it with spirit and peanut oil equally. Cook the honey until it is done. Put the mash of jujubes and sweet almond along with honey in the jar, and then heat it over a slow fire until it nearly boils. Put the juice of rehmanniae root after it cools. Seal the mouth of the jar for 7 days. Shake the jar once daily.

**Directions**  Take 10 ml twice daily.

**Indications**  Incoordination between spleen and stomach manifested by constipation, anorexia, cough with little sputum.

**Recipe** 11

**Ingredients**

Radix et Rhizoma Rhei, 30 g

Natrii Sulphas, 10 g

spirit, 100 g

**Process**  Pound rhubarb into pieces and grind sodium sulphate into fine powder. Decoct the two ingredients with spirit until 50 ml left. Remove the dregs for later use.

**Directions**  Take the decoction once daily.

**Indications**  Constipation accompanied by distending pain in the abdomen. Contraindicated for senile and pregnant cases.

**Recipe** 12

**Ingredients**

Mel, 500 g

distiller's yeast, 50 g

**Process**. Add 1000 ml of water in the honey. Grind distiller's yeast into powder and mix it with honey equally. Seal the container for 45 days and then remove the dregs for later use.

**Directions** Take 10 ml twice daily.

**Indications** Senile constipation, cough due to deficiency of lung qi.

**Recipe** 13

**Ingredients**

Fructus Mori, 1000 g

Semen Oryzae Glutinosae, 500 g

**Process** Wash the mulberries clean and pound them to extract juice. Mix the juice with polished glutinous rice to make wine.

**Directions** Take right amount of such wine thre e times daily.

**Indication** Senile constipation.

**Recipe** 14

**Ingredients**

Semen Sesami Nigrum

**Process** Wash black sesame seed clean and steam for three times. Then cook them until they are done. Grind the seed into fine powder. Mix right amount of Mel to make pills. Each weighs 10 g.

**Directions** Take one pill with warm millet wine twice daily.

**Indication** Chronic constipation.

**Recipe** 15

**Ingredients**

Semen Juglandis, 100 g

white sugar, 50 g

millet wine, 100 ml

**Process** Put walnut kernels along with sugar and millet wine in an earthenware pot. Decoct the ingredients over a strong fire. Then let it boil over a slow fire for 10 minutes.

**Directions** Take the decoction once or twice daily. One course consisting of 10 days.

**Indication** Habitual constipation.

## Section 18 Angina Pectoris

Angina pectoris is characterized by pain in the centre of the chest, which is induced by exercise and relieved by rest and may spread to the jaws and arms. Angina pectoris occurs when the demand for blood by the heart exceeds the supply of the coronary arteries and it usually results from coronary artery heart atheroma. It is known as "Xiongbi" or "Zhenxintong" in traditional Chinese medicine. It is mostly caused by constitutional deficiency of either heart qi or heart yang, leading to invasion of pathogenic cold. Cold retention in the interior and stagnation of qi due to cold retention cause obstruction of the channels and collaterals. Impairment of the spleen and stomach due to improper diet such as over indulgence of sweet, greasy, raw or cold food can cause accumulation of phlegm-damp obstructing the chest yang. However, prolonged stagnation of qi due to emotional disturbance cause poor blood circulation. And stasis of blood in the vessels results in the condition.

**Recipe 1**
**Ingredients**
Ganoderma Lucidum, 30 g
Radix Salviae Miltiorrhizae, 5 g
Radix Notoginseng, 5 g
spirits, 500 ml
**Process** Soak lucid ganoderma, Dan-Shen root and notoginseng in spirit and seal the container, put it in a cool, dry place for 15 days. Shake the container once daily during soaking. Filter the tincture and store it up for future administration.
**Directions** Take 5 ml once daily.
**Indication** Angina pectoris.

**Recipe 2**
**Ingredients**
Cortex Moutan Radicis, 30 g
Radix Notoginseng, 10 g
Rhizoma Chuanxiong, 10 g
spirit, 1000 ml
**Process** Soak moutan bark, notoginseng and szechuan lovage rhizome in spirit and seal the container, put it in a cool, dry place for two months. Shake the container once daily during soaking. Filter the tincture and store it up for future administration.
**Directions** Take 15 ml before sleep daily.
**Indication** Angina pectoris.

**Recipe 3**
**Ingredients**
Bulbus Allii Macrostemi, 15 g
Fructus Trichosanthis, 20 g
spirit, 15 ml
water, 200 ml
**Process** Decoct macrostem onion, snakegourd fruit and spirit in 200 ml of water over fire until there is 100 ml of the decoction left.

**Directions**  Take 50 ml of the decoction twice daily.
**Indication**  Angina pectoris.

**Recipe** 4
**Ingredients**
Radix Salviae Miltiorrhizae, 50-100 g
spirit, 1000 ml
**Process**  Grind Dan-Shen root into powder and soak the powder in spirit and seal the container, put it in a cool, dry place for 15 days. Shake the container once daily during soaking. Filter the tincture and store it up for future administration.
**Directions**  Take 20-30 ml three times daily.
**Indication**  Angina pectoris.

**Recipe** 5
**Ingredients**
Radix Polygoni Multiflori, 60 ml
spirit, 500 ml
**Process**  Cut fleeceflower root into pieces and soak them in spirit and seal the container, put it in a cool, dry place for 5 days. Shake the container once daily during soaking. Filter the tincture and store it up for future administration.
**Directions**  Take 10 to 15 ml once or twice daily.
**Indication**  Arteriosclerosis.

## Section 19 Hypertension

Hypertension refers to elevation of the arterial blood pressure above the normal range expected in a particular age group. Arterial pressure fluctuates in most persons, whether they are normotensive or hypertensive. The definitions should consider not only the level of diastolic pressure but also systolic pressure, age, sex, and race. Those who are classified as having labile hypertension are patients who sometimes but not always have arterial pressures within the hypertensive range. These patients are often considered to have borderline hypertension. Sustained hypertension can become accelerated or enter a malignant phase. Though a patient with malignant hypertension often has a blood pressure above 200/140, it is papilledema, usually accompanied by retinal hemorrhages and exudates, and not the absolute pressure level, that defines this condition. Accelerated hypertension signifies a significant recent increase over previous hypertensive levels associated with evidence of vascular damages on funduscopic examination but without papilledema.

The cause of elevated arterial pressure is unknown in most cases. Patients with arterial hypertension and no definable cause are said to have primary, essential, or idiopathic hypertension. By definition, the underlying mechanism(s) is unknown; however, the kidney probably plays a central role. There are characteristics common to many patients in this group, however including a positive family history for hypertension and evidence for increased vascular reactivity. Genetic factors have long been assumed to be important in the genesis of hypertension. A number of environmental factors have been specifically implicated in the development of hypertension including salt intake, obesity, occupation, family size, and crowding. These factors have all been assumed to be important in the increase in blood pressure with age in more affluent societies, in contrast to the decline in blood pressure with age in more primitive cultures. Age, race, sex, smoking, serum cholesterol, glucose intolerance, weight, and perhaps renin activity may all alter the prognosis of essential hypertension.

Secondary hypertension embraces mainly renal and endocrine types. It may also result from diseases of the arteries (such as coarctation of the aorta) or other various kinds of diseases.

This condition belongs to the categories of Headache and Dizziness. It is mostly caused by abnormal ascending of liver fire; deficiency of both liver yin and kidney yin; hyperactivity of liver yang due to deficiency of yin.

**Recipe** 1
**Ingredients**
Cortex Eucommiae, 30 g

spirit, 500 ml

**Process**  Soak eucommia bark in spirits and seal the container, put it in a cool, dry place for 7 days. Shake the container once daily during soaking. Filter the tincture and store it up for future administration.

**Directions**  Take 10 to 20 ml twice or three times daily.

**Indication**  Hypertension.

**Recipe** 2
**Ingredients**
Rhizoma Polygonati, 50 g

Radix Polygoni Multiflori, 30 g

Fructus Lycii, 30 g

spirit, 1000 ml

**Process**  Soak barbary wolfberry fruit, siberian solomonseal rhizome and fleeceflower root in spirit and seal the container for, put it in a cool, dry place 7 days. Shake the container once daily during soaking. Filter the tincture and store it up for future administration.

**Directions**  Take 10 ml before meals.

**Indication**  Hypertension.

**Recipe** 3
**Ingredients**
Flos Chrysanthemi, 10 g

polished glutinous rice wine, 50 ml

**Process**  Cut chrysanthemum flower into pieces and then mix them with rice wine. Decoct the mixture over fire until it boils.

**Directions**  Take the decoction twice daily.

**Indication**  Dizziness due to hypertension of lung-heat type.

## Section 20 Hyperlipemia

Hyperlipemia refers to the presence in the blood of an abnormally high concentration of fats. It belongs to the categories of "Yu zheng" (blood stasis) and "Tan zhuo" (stagnation of phlegm) in TCM. A commonly encountered type is, namely, deficiency of spleen to send up essential substances with thick phlegm accumulated in the interior, which manifested mainly by drowsy heaviness in the head, sensation of stuffiness in the chest and abdomen, or nausea, or a full figure with dyspnea, heaviness sensation in the body, numbness and heaviness of the limbs, white greasy or moist coating on the tongue, and taut and slippery pulse.

**Recipe**
**Ingredients**
Fructus Crataegi, 300 g
Fructus Jujubae, 30 g
brown sugar, 30 g
rice wine, 1000 ml

**Process**  Soak jujubes, hawthorn fruit and brown sugar in rice wine and seal the container, put it in a cool, dry place for 10 days. Shake the container once daily during soaking. Filter the tincture and store it up for future administration.

**Directions**  Take 30 to 60 ml before sleep.

**Indication**  Hyperlipemia. Contraindicated for cases with constipation of sthenic-heat type.

## Section 21 Hypotension

Hypotension refers to a condition in which the arterial blood pressure is abnormally low. It occurs after excessive fluid loss (e. g. through diarrhea, burns, or vomiting) or following severe blood loss (hemorrhage) from any cause. Other causes embrace myocardial infarction, pulmonary embolism, severe infections, allergic reactions, arrhythmias, acute abdominal conditions (e. g. pancreatitis), Addison's disease, and drugs (e. g. an overdose of the drugs used to treat hypertension. Some people experience orthostatic hypotension. Chronic hypotension is mainly considered in this section.

Patients with true chronic hypotension may complain of lethargy, weakness, easy fatigability, and dizziness or faintness, especially if arterial pressure is lowered further when the erect position is assumed. These symptoms are presumably due to a decrease in perfusion of the brain, heart, skeletal muscle, and other organs. Chronic hypotension occasionally results from severe reduction of the cardiac output. The major endocrine causes of chronic hypotension are associated with deficient gluco- and mineralocorticoid secretion and resultant reductions of the intravascular and interstitial fluid volume. Hypotension is usually more pronounced in patients with primary adrenocortical insufficiency than in those with hypopituitarism because secretion of the salt-retaining adrenocortical hormone aldosterone is partially preserved in pituitary insufficiency. Malnutrition, cachexia, chronic bed rest, and a variety of neurologic disorders may result in chronic hypotension, especially in the standing position. Multiple sclerosis, amyotrophic lateral sclerosis, syringomyelia, syphilitic or diabetic tabes dorsalis, peripheral neuropathies, spinal cord section, diabetic neuropathy, extensive lumbodorsal sympathectomy, and the administration of drugs interfering with nerve transmission in the sympathetic nervous system are all associated with orthostatic hypotension.

The subsequent prescription are effective for chronic hypotension manifested by vertigo and other deficiency syndromes.

### Recipe 1
**Ingredients**
Radix Ginseng, 100 g
Pericarpium Citri Reticulatae, 2 g
Rhizoma Zingiberis, 2 g
Fructus Jujubae, 2 g
spirit, 1000 ml

**Process**  Soak ginseng, tangerine peel, fresh ginger and jujube in spirits, seal the container and put it in a cool, dry place for 3 to 6 months. Shake the container once daily during soaking. Filter the tincture and store it up for future administration.

**Directions**  Take 5 ml once or twice daily.
**Indication**  Hypotension.

### Recipe 2
**Ingredients**
grape wine
**Directions**  Take right amount of wine once daily.
**Indication**  Hypotension.

## Section 22 Anemia

Anemia refers to a reduction in the quantity of the oxygen- carrying pigment hemoglobin in the blood. The main symptoms are excessive tiredness and fatigability, breathlessness on exertion, pallor, and poor resistance to infection. There are many causes of anemia. It may be due to loss of blood, or from chronic bleeding. Iron-deficiency anemia, macrocytic anemia, hemolytic anemia, aplastic anemia are the main,secondary anemias. This condition belongs to "Xuexu" (blood deficiency), "Xulao" (consumptive disease) and "Xuhuang" (sallow complexion of insufficiency type) in traditional Chinese medicine. It is mostly caused by deficiency of the heart, spleen, qi and blood; deficiency of liver yin, kidney yin, essence and blood; deficiency of both blood and qi with insufficiency of spleen yang and kidney yang.

### Recipe 1
**Ingredients**
Colla Corii Asini, 15 g
polished glutinous rice, 50 g
Mel, 30 g
rice wine, 15-20 ml

**Process**  Put polished glutinous rice into water. Cook the rice into gruel. Add donkey-hide gelatin and honey into the gruel and mix them equally.

**Directions**  Take the gruel when it is warm, three times daily. Ten days consisted of one course.

**Indication**  Anemia.

### Recipe 2
**Ingredients**
Arillus Longan, 250 g
Radix Polygoni Multiflori, 250 g
Caulis Spatholobi, 250 g
rice wine, 1500 ml

**Process**  Soak longan aril, fleeceflower root and suberect spatholobus stem in rice wine and seal the container, put it in a cool, dry place for 10 days. Shake the container once daily during soaking. Filter the tincture and store it up for future administration.

**Directions**  Take 15 to 30 g twice daily.

**Indication**  Anemia.

## Section 23 Edema

Edema refers to retention of fluid in the body, resulting in the puffiness of the head, face, eyelids, limbs, abdomen and even the general body. The condition elaborated here comprises the edema caused by acute and chronic nephritis, congestive heart failure, endocrinal disease and dystrophy in modern medicine. Edema of yang-type is mostly due to wading through water or being caught in rain, exposure to cold after bath, invasion of pathogenic heat into the interior due to furuncle effect. These factors may cause dysfunction of the lung in dispersing and descending, and that of the spleen in transforming and transporting, leading to eventual retention of pathogenic damp-water flooding over body superficies. Edema of yin-type is often due to improper diet, deficiency of spleen qi, impairment of kidney and spleen results in poor transforming and transporting, and internal retention of damp-water. The deficiency of kidney leads to poor water metabolism and failure of kidney to control over urination, resulting in flooding of damp-water to the exterior of the body.

**Recipe** 1
**Ingredients**
carp, 1
rice wine, 1500 ml
**Process** Cook carp in rice wine over a slow fire until it is done.
**Directions** Take right amount of fish three times daily.
**Indication** Anasarca.

**Recipe** 2
**Ingredients**
finless eel, 150 g
garlic, 10 g
spirit, 15 ml
**Process** Cook finless eel along with garlic and spirit until they are done.
**Directions** Take right amount of fish three times daily.
**Indication** Edema of the abdomen.

**Recipe** 3
**Ingredients**
quail, 2
spirit, 20 g
**Process** Skin the roaster and get rid of the entrails of the quails, put them in an earthenware pot with 20 g of spirit and a right amount of water; stew it over slow fire until it is done.
**Directions** Eat the quails once daily. One course consisting of 7 days.

**Indication**  Nephrogenic edema.

**Recipe** 4
**Ingredients**
soya beans, 250 g
rice wine
**Process**  Add 1000 ml of water in soya beans and decoct them over fire until 250 ml of the decoction is left.
**Directions**  Take 80 ml of the decoction along with right amount of rice wine three times daily.
**Indication**  Nutritional edema.

**Recipe** 5
**Ingredients**
peanut, 100 g
carp, 1
spirit
**Process**  Put peanuts and carp in an earthenware pot with a right amount of water; stew it over slow fire until it is done.
**Directions**  Take the peanuts and fish along with right amount of spirit once daily.
**Indications**  Nutritional edema accompanied by general weakness, diuresis, dizziness and dyspnea.

**Recipe** 6
**Ingredients**
black soya beans, 200 g
spirit, 500 ml
**Process**  Decoct soya beans along with 1000 ml of water over slow fire until there is 500 ml left. Add 500 ml of spirit in the decoction and decoct the mixture over slow fire until 500 ml left.
**Directions**  Take the 500/3 ml of the decoction when it is warm, three times daily.
**Indication**  Anasarca.

**Recipe** 7
**Ingredients**
Semen Coicis, 60 g
spirit, 500 ml
**Process**  Clean the coix seed and fill them in a gauze bag, fasten the bag. Soak the bag in 500 ml of spirit and seal the container, put it in a cool, dry place for 7 days. Shake the container once daily during soaking. Filter the tincture and store it up for future administration.
**Directions**  Take 5 ml before sleep daily.
**Indication**  Edema of the lower extremities.

**Recipe** 8
**Ingredients**

Fructus Mori, 100 g

spirit, 500 ml

**Process**  Wash the mulberries clean and extract their juice. Soak the dregs in 500 ml of spirit along with the juice and seal the container, put it in a cool, dry place for 3 days. Shake the container once daily during soaking. Filter the tincture and store it up for future administration.

**Directions**  Take 5 ml twice daily.

**Indication**  Edema of the lower extremities.

**Recipe** 9
**Ingredients**

Rhizoma Polygonati, 20 g

spirit, 500 ml

**Process**  Wash siberian Solomonseal rhizome clean and cut into pieces. Fill them in a gauze bag and then fasten the mouth. Soak it in spirit and seal the container, put it in a cool, dry place for 30 days. Shake the container once daily during soaking. Filter the tincture and store it up for future administration.

**Directions**  Take 5 ml twice daily.

**Indication**  Edema of the face.

## Section 24 Paruria

Paruria, embracing frequency of micturition, diuresis, oliguria etc., is considered to be concerned with urinary infection, prostatitis, diabetes mellitus, and dysfunction of hypothalamo-hypophyseal system. According to traditional Chinese medicine, paruria is the consequence of poor function of lower jiao and dysfunction of the urinary bladder in controlling urination due to weak constitution and kidney qi deficiency. Insufficiency of kidney qi in the aged or impairment of the kidney due to over sexual indulgence may also cause incontinence of urine because of cold retention in the lower jiao and poor opening function of the urinary bladder. Internal injuries due to seven emotional disturbances such as fear, fright and over thinking affecting the spleen and lung can cause deficiency of them. And the superior deficiency cannot control the inferior so that the urinary bladder will lose its control over urinary discharge. Accumulation of damp-heat that flows down to the urinary bladder leads to paruria. Moreover, blood stasis due to various reasons obstructing in the urinary bladder will cause the dysfunction of urinary bladder in transporting qi. Therefore paruria occurs because the urinary bladder does not control urination.

**Recipe 1**
**Ingredients**
Sulphur, 6 g
Bulbus Allii, 12 g
spirits, right amount
**Process** Grind sulphur and dried Chinese green onion into fine powder and then mix it with spirits. Apply the mixture on Shenque(RN8) and other points on the lower abdomen. Heat these points with moxa sticks.
**Directions** Apply moxibustion twice daily.
**Indication** Enuresis.

**Recipe 2**
**Ingredients**
Semen Allii Tuberosi, 6 g
spirits, right amount
water, right amount
**Process** Grind Chinese chive seed into fine powder.
**Directions** Take the powder with right amount of spirits and water once daily.
**Indication** Frequency of micturition.

**Recipe 3**
**Ingredients**
Semen Juglandis, 30 g
rice wine, 30 ml
**Directions** Take the walnut kernel with warm rice wine before sleep once daily. One course consisting of 5 days.
**Indication** Diuresis due to deficiency of kidney qi.

**Recipe 4**
**Ingredients**
Radix Glycyrrhizae, 9 g
Radix Euphorbiae Kansui, 9 g
white spirits, right amount
**Process** Grind liquorice and kansui root into fine powder. Mix it with hot spirits.
**Directions** Apply the mixture on Shenque(RN8) and heat the point with moxa sticks, once daily.
**Indication** Uroschesis.

**Recipe 5**
**Ingredients**

Semen Coicis, 60 g

white spirits, 500 ml

**Process**  Wash coix seed clean and fill them in a gauze bag with the mouth of the bag fastened. Soak the bag in spirits and seal the container for 7 days.

**Directions**  Take 30 ml once daily.

**Indication**  Oliguria.

## Recipe 6
**Ingredients**

Semen Sinapis Albae, 10 g

spirits, right amount

**Process**  Grind white mustard seed into powder and then mix it with spirits.

**Directions**  Apply the mixture on Shenque(RN8) and heat the point with moxa sticks, once daily.

**Indications**  Dysuria and constipation.

## Recipe 7
**Ingredients**

Fructus Mori, 100 g

spirits, 500 ml

**Process**  Wash mulberries clean and pound them to extract their juice. Fill a gauze bag with the juice and fasten the mouth. Soak the bag in spirits and seal the container for 3 days.

**Directions**  Take 10 ml three times daily.

**Indication**  Dysuria.

## Recipe 8
**Ingredients**

Folium Sacchari, 30 g

spirits, right amount

**Process**  Decoct the sugar cane leaves with spirits.

**Directions**  Take the decoction once daily.

**Indications**  Stranguria due to disorder of qi manifested by slow and painful discharge of urine, urgency of urination.

## Recipe 9
**Ingredients**

Rhizoma Nelumbinis Recens, 60 g

Herba Plantaginis, 60 g

spirits, right amount

**Process**  Pound lotus root and plantain herb into mash to extract juice. Decoct the juice with right amount of spirits.

**Directions**  Take 5 ml of the decoction twice daily.
**Indication**  Dysuria.

**Recipe** 10
**Ingredients**
pork bladder, 1
millet wine, right amount
**Process**  Bake the pork bladder and then grind it into fine powder.
**Directions**  Take the powder with right amount of warm millet wine.
**Indications**  Dysuria, vesical tenesmus.

**Recipe** 11
**Ingredients**
Gecko, 2
millet wine, 500 ml
**Process**  Remove the heads, feet and scales of the geckoes and then soak them in millet wine and seal the container for 7 days.
**Directions**  Take 5 to 10 ml twice daily.
**Indication**  Frequency of micturition. Contraindicated for cases with cough due to suffering from wind and cold evil.

**Recipe** 12
**Ingredients**
Rhizoma Anemarrhenae, 60 g
Cortex Phellodendri, 60 g
Cortex Cinnamomi, 4 g
Mel, right amount
spirits, right amount
**Process**  Stir-fry common anemarrhena rhizomes, cassia bark and phellodendron bark with right amount of spirits and then grind into powder. Mix it with right amount of Mel to make pills the size of a Chinese parasol fruit.
**Directions**  Take 50 pills with warm water, twice daily.
**Indication**  Dysuria due to damp-heat in the lower jiao.

**Recipe** 13
**Ingredients**
Crinis Carbonisatus, 7.5 g
Eupolyphaga seu Steleophaga, 7
spirit, right amount

water, right amount

**Process** Pound carbonized hair and ground beetles into mash. Soak it in spirits and water for 7 days. Remove the dregs for later use.

**Directions** Take the tincture once daily.

**Indication** Dysuria.

## Section 25 Nephritis

Nephritis is divided into acute and chronic types, both of which are clinically characterized by edema, proteinuria and hypertension. Acute nephritis in most cases belongs to the categories of "Fengshui" (wind edema) and "Yangshui" (yang-type edema); while chronic nephritis in most cases belongs to the category of "Zhengshui" (anasarca with shortness of breath), "Shishui" (stony edema) and "Yinshui" (yin-type edema). Acute nephritis is mainly due to 1) attack of wind-cold to the lung and stagnation of qi in Sanjiao; 2) retention of wind-heat in the lung and accumulation of dampness and toxic materials and 3) toxic heat attacking the interior causing damage to the yin blood. While chronic nephritis is mostly due to 1) overflow of water in the body due to insufficiency of both the spleen-yang and the kidney-yang; insufficiency of both the spleen and the kidney with deficiency of essence and blood and 3) hyperactivity of the liver yang due to deficiency of both liver yin and kidney yin. The following prescriptions can applied for alleviating the symptoms.

**Recipe 1**

**Ingredients**

Semen Luffae, 9 g

millet wine, right amount

**Process** Bake the seed of luffa and then grind into powder.

**Directions** Take the powder with warm millet wine once daily.

**Indication** Pyelonephritis.

**Recipe 2**

**Ingredients**

flesh of soft shelled turtle, 500 g

Bulbus Allii, 60 g

white sugar, right amount

plain spirits, right amount

**Process** Cook the flesh of soft-shelled turtle with garlic, white sugar, plain spirits and right amount of water over a slow fire.

**Directions** Take 500/3 g of the flesh three times daily.

**Indication** Chronic nephritis.

**Recipe** 3
**Ingredients**
Semen Juglandis, 9 g
Periostracum Serpentis, 1
millet wine, right amount
**Process** Grind dried walnut kernel and snake slough into fine powder.
**Directions** Take the powder with warm millet wine once daily.
**Indication** Nephritis.

## Section 26 Renal Tuberculosis

Tuberculosis is a necrotizing bacterial infection with protean manifestations and wide distribution. Second to the upper lobes of the lungs, the kidney is the most common site for the late appearance of localized tuberculous infection. The mechanism of implantation is the same as that in the pulmonary apexes, namely, by hematogenous spread early in the infection. The oxygen tension in thee cortical portion of the kidney approaches that in arterial blood, which enhances the growth and persistence of tubercle bacilli. As in the lungs, foci of tuberculosis may remain dormant for many years and produce clinical disease late in life. The pathologic process is the same as in the lung: inflammation, followed by caseation, liquefaction, and discharge of contaminated material into the collecting system and down the ureter to the bladder and, in men, to the genital tract.

Symptoms of renal tuberculosis are usually insidious and may be overlooked completely until the appearance of cystitis or epididymitis. Gross or microscopic hematuria and pyuria with a "sterile" urine on culture for bacteria should always call tuberculosis to mind and lead to the performance of a tuberculin skin test and culture of urine for tubercle bacilli. Intravenous pyelography may reveal a cortical cavity communicating with the calyceal system. Symptoms usually subside promptly with chemotherapy. Resection of residual areas of destruction is only rarely necessary.

**Recipe**
**Ingredients**
Herba Portulacae, 1500 g
millet wine, 1250 ml
**Process** Wash portulaca clean and then pound into mash. Soak the mash in millet wine and seal the container, put it in a cool, dry place for 3 to 4 days. Shake the container once daily during soaking. Filter the tincture and store it up for future administration.
**Directions** Take 15 to 20 ml three times daily.
**Indication** Renal tuberculosis.

## Section 27 Impotency

Impotency refers to weakness of penis erecting during sexual intercourse, characterized by poor erecting or erection that lasts only for seconds. It may be manifested in various ways: loss of desire, inability to obtain or maintain an erection, premature ejaculation, absence of emission, inability to achieve orgasm. It is often the consequence of deficiency of the essential qi and decline of life gate fire due to over sexual indulgence or juvenile masturbation. Over consumption of qi of the heart, spleen and kidney due to fear, fright or worry can also cause impotency. Internal damp-heat retention affecting the liver and kidney with looseness of penis accounts for another factor to cause impotency.

### Recipe 1
**Ingredients**
the penis and testicle of a male sika deer or red deer, one set
Cornu Cervi Pantotrichum, 30 g
Gecko, 2
plain spirits, 1000 ml
**Process** Soak the deer's penis and testicle, pilose antler and geckoes in plain spirits and seal the container, put it in a cool, dry place for one week. Shake the container once daily during soaking. Filter the tincture and store it up for future administration.
**Directions** Take 30 ml twice daily.
**Indication** Impotency.

### Recipe 2
**Ingredients**
Herba Cistanchis, 30 g
plain spirits, 500 ml
**Process** Soak desertliving cistanche in plain spirits and seal the container, put it in a cool, dry place for one week. Shake the container once daily during soaking. Filter the tincture and store it up for future administration.
**Directions** Take 10 ml twice daily.
**Indication** Impotency.

### Recipe 3
**Ingredients**
Cordyceps, 100 g
Herba Saussureae Involucratae, 60 g

plain spirits, 200 ml

**Process**  Soak the snow lotus herb and Chinese caterpillar fungus in plain spirits and seal the container, put it in a cool, dry place for one week. Shake the container once daily during soaking. Filter the tincture and store it up for future administration.

**Directions**  Take 10 ml twice daily.

**Indications**  Impotency, emission.

### Recipe 4
**Ingredients**

Gecko, 2

millet wine, 500 ml

**Process**  Remove the heads, feet and scales of the geckoes, and soak them in millet wine and seal the container, put it in a cool, dry place for one week. Shake the container once daily during soaking. Filter the tincture and store it up for future administration.

**Directions**  Take 5 ml twice daily.

**Indication**  Impotency due to deficiency of kidney.

### Recipe 5
**Ingredients**

Herba Cynomorii, 30 g

plain spirits, 500 ml

**Process**  Soak the cynomorium horn in plain spirits and seal the container, put it in a cool, dry place for one week. Shake the container once daily during soaking. Filter the tincture and store it up for future administration.

**Directions**  Take 20 ml twice daily.

**Indication**  Impotency due to deficiency of kidney.

### Recipe 6
**Ingredients**

Herba Epimedii, 30 g

plain spirits, 500 ml

**Process**  Soak the epimedium in plain spirits and seal the container, put it in a cool, dry place for one week. Shake the container once daily during soaking. Filter the tincture and store it up for future administration.

**Directions**  Take 20 to 30 ml twice or three times daily.

**Indication**  Impotency due to deficiency of kidney.

### Recipe 7
**Ingredients**

Rhizoma Curculiginis, 240 g

spirits, 1500 ml

**Process** Soak the curculigo rhizome in plain spirits and seal the container, put it in a cool, dry place for 3 days. Shake the container once daily during soaking. Filter the tincture and store it up for future administration.

**Directions** Take 30 to 60 ml twice daily.

**Indication** Impotency.

**Recipe** 8

**Ingredients**

Radix Ginseng, 100 g

Pericarpium Citri Reticulatae, 20 g

Rhizoma Zingiberis, 20 g

Fructus Jujubae, 20 g

plain spirits, 500 ml

**Process** Soak the ginseng, tangerine peel, ginger and jujubes in plain spirits and seal the container, put it in a cool, dry place for three to six months. Shake the container once daily during soaking. Filter the tincture and store it up for future administration.

**Directions** Take 5 ml once or twice daily.

**Indication** Impotency.

**Recipe** 9

**Ingredients**

Radix Morindae Officinalis, 30 g

Radix Achyranthis Bidentatae, 30 g

plain spirits, 500 ml

**Process** Soak the morinda root and achyranthes root in plain spirits and seal the container, put it in a cool, dry place for 7 days. Shake the container once daily during soaking. Filter the tincture and store it up for future administration.

**Directions** Take 10 to 20 ml twice daily.

**Indication** Impotency due to deficiency of kidney.

**Recipe** 10

**Ingredients**

Carassius Auratus, 1

plain spirits, 50 ml

**Process** Remove the internal organs and scrape the scales off the crucian carp. Wash it clean and put it in an earthenware pot. Add spirits and a right amount of water in the pot and cook the fish until it is done.

**Directions** Take the fish and soup once other day.

**Indication** Impotency.

**Recipe** 11
**Ingredients**
Passer Montanus Saturatus, 3
Semen Cuscutae, 15 g
Herba Cistanchis, 15 g
rice wine, 1000 ml

**Process**   Remove the feathers and internal organs of the sparrows and wash them clean. Soak dodder seed and desertliving cistanche along with sparrows in rice wine and seal the container, put it in a cool, dry place for 7 days. Remove the sparrows from the tincture and store it up for future administration.

**Directions**   Take 10 ml twice daily.

**Indication**   Impotency due to deficiency of kidney.

**Recipe** 12
**Ingredients**
Fructus Foenicuii, 30 g
Macrobrachium Nipponense, 90 g
millet wine, right amount

**Process**   Stir-fry the common fennel fruit and grind into fine powder. Pound the shrimps into mash and mix it with the powder equally to make pills. Each pill weighs 3 g.

**Directions**   Take one pill with a right amount of millet wine twice daily.

**Indication**   Impotency, soreness and weakness of the waist and lower extremities due to deficiency of kidney qi.

**Recipe** 13
**Ingredients**
Semen Juglandis, 1
Semen Allii Tuberosi, 6 g
millet wine, right amount

**Process**   Make decoction with Chinese chive seed and walnut kernel in a right amount of water.

**Directions**   Take half of the decoction with millet wine twice daily. One course consists of 3 days.

**Indication**   Impotency, emission.

**Recipe** 14
**Ingredients**
Canis Familiaris, 1
millet wine, right amount

**Process**   Bake the penis and testicle of a dog and then grind them into fine powder.

**Directions**  Take 3 to 4 g with millet wine twice daily.
**Indication**  Impotency.

**Recipe** 15
**Ingredients**
Semen Momordicae Charantia, 150 g
millet wine, right amount
**Process**  Stir-fry the seed of balsam pear until they are done. Grind the seed into fine powder.
**Directions**  Take 15 g of the powder with millet wine, three times daily. One course consists of 10 days.
**Indication**  Impotency.

**Recipe** 16
**Ingredients**
Fructus Litchi, 500 g
rice wine, 1000 ml
**Process**  Soak the litchi fruit in rice wine and seal the container, put it in a cool, dry place for 7 days. Shake the container once daily during soaking. Filter the tincture and store it up for future administration.
**Directions**  Take 30 ml twice daily.
**Indication**  Impotency.

**Recipe** 17
**Ingredients**
Herba Allii Tuberosi, 150 g
dried shelled shrimps, 150 g
egg, 1
vegetable oil, right amount
plain spirits, 50 ml
**Process**  Stir-fry dried shelled shrimps, Chinese chives and egg in a right amount of vegetable oil in a pot until they are done.
**Directions**  Take the food with spirits, once daily. One course consists of ten days.
**Indication**  Impotency.

**Recipe** 18
**Ingredients**
Semen Allii Tuberosi, 500 g
rice wine, 2500 ml
**Process**  Soak the Chinese chive seed in rice wine and seal the container, put it in a cool, dry place for one week. Shake the container once daily during soaking. Filter the tincture and store it up

for future administration.

**Directions**   Take 20 ml twice daily.

**Indication**   Impotency, premature ejaculation.

**Recipe** 19

**Ingredients**

Cortex Acanthopanacis Radicis, 40 g

plain spirits, 1000 ml

**Process**   Soak the acanthopanax bark in plain spirits and seal the container, put it in a cool, dry place for one week. Shake the container once daily during soaking. Filter the tincture and store it up for future administration.

**Directions**   Take 5 ml three times daily.

**Indication**   Impotency.

**Recipe** 20

**Ingredients**

Semen Gossypii, 30 g

rice wine, right amount

**Process**   Stir-fry the cotton seed until they are done. Remove the shells of the seed.

**Directions**   Take 3 g of the seed (take one's time chewing the seed) with rice wine, twice daily.

**Indication**   Impotency, thinness of seminal fluid.

**Recipe** 21

**Ingredients**

Fructus Rubi, 50 g

Semen Allii Tuberosi, 50 g

plain spirits, right amount

**Process**   Soak raspberries, Chinese chive seed in plain spirits and seal the container, put it in a cool, dry place for 3 days. Take the dregs out and bake them. Grind the dried mulberries and Chinese chive seed into fine powder, store it up for future administration.

**Directions**   Take 15 g of the powder, twice daily.

**Indication**   Impotency.

**Recipe** 22

**Ingredients**

Macrobrachium Nipponense, 200 g

plain spirits, 250 ml

**Process**   Soak the fresh river shrimps in plain spirits and seal the container, put it in a cool, dry place for 7 days. Shake the container once daily during soaking. Filter the tincture and store it up for future administration.

**Directions**  Take 10 ml three times daily. Cook the shrimps and eat them when the spirits is drunk up.

**Indication**  Impotency. Contraindicated for cases with syndrome of deficiency of yin.

## Recipe 23
**Ingredients**

Cornu Cervi Pantotrichum, 10 g

Rhizoma Dioscoreae, 30 g

plain spirits, 500 ml

**Process**  Cut the pilose antler into thin slices and soak them along with Chinese yams in plain spirits and seal the container, put it in a cool, dry place for 7 days. Shake the container once daily during soaking. Filter the tincture and store it up for future administration.

**Directions**  Take 10 ml before meals three times daily.

**Indications**  Impotency, thinness of seminal fluid, premature ejaculation, spermatorrhea.

## Recipe 24
**Ingredients**

Cornu Cervi Pantotrichum, 2 g

Fructus Lycii, 60 g

Radix Ginseng, 10 g

Hippocampus, 3 g

plain spirits, 1500 ml

**Process**  Soak pilose antler, wolfberry fruit, ginseng and sea horse in plain spirits and seal the container, put it in a cool, dry place for 30 days. Shake the container once daily during soaking. Filter the tincture and store it up for future administration.

**Directions**  Take 20 ml at bed time, daily.

**Indication**  Impotency.

## Recipe 25
**Ingredients**

Radix Morindae Officinalis, 25 g

Semen Cuscutae, 25 g

plain spirits, 500 ml

**Process**  Soak morinda root and dodder seed in plain spirits and seal the container, put it in a cool, dry place for 7 days. Shake the container once daily during soaking. Filter the tincture and store it up for future administration.

**Directions**  Take 10 ml twice daily.

**Indications**  Impotency, frequency of micturition.

**Recipe** 26
**Ingredients**
Peni et Testes Callorhini, one set
Radix Ginseng, 15 g
plain spirits, 1000 ml

**Process**  Cut the ursine seal's penis and testes into slices and soak them along with ginseng in plain spirits and seal the container, put it in a cool, dry place for 10 days. Shake the container once daily during soaking. Filter the tincture and store it up for future administration.

**Directions**  Take 10 ml twice daily.

**Indications'**  Impotency, thinness of seminal fluid, listlessness, lassitude and fatigue, premature ejaculation due to deficiency of kidney yang.

## Section 28   Premature Ejaculation

This disorder seldom has an organic cause. It is usually related to anxiety in the sexual situation, unreasonable expectations about performance, or an emotional disorder. The following prescriptions are effective for this condition in considerable degrees.

**Recipe** 1
**Ingredients**
Fructus Rosae Laevigatae, 500 g
Radix Codonopsis Pilosulae, 50 g
Radix Dipsaci, 50 g
Herba Epimedii, 50 g
Fructus Cnidii, 50 g
plain spirits, 2500 ml

**Process**  Soak the above ingredients in plain spirits and seal the container, put it in a cool, dry place for 15 days. Shake the container once daily during soaking. Filter the tincture and store it up for future administration.

**Directions**  Take 25 ml twice daily.

**Indication**  Premature ejaculation.

**Recipe** 2
**Ingredients**
Herba Allii Tuberosi, 200 g
Lumbricus, 50 g

millet wine, 100 ml

**Process** Cut open the earthworms and wash them clean. Extract the Chinese chives to get juice. Mix earthworms with the juice and pound into mash. Put the mash in boiling millet wine for 5 minutes. Then keep the container away from fire and seal it for 10 minutes.

**Directions** Take all of the tincture once daily. One course consists of 3 days.

**Indication** Premature ejaculation.

**Recipe** 3
**Ingredients**
Rhizoma Smilacis Glabrae, 50 g
pork, 100 g
millet wine, 50 ml

**Process** Put smilax glabra rhizome and pork and millet wine in an earthenware pot and put in a right amount of water. Cook them over a slow fire for two hours.

**Directions** Take half of the meat and soup twice daily.

**Indication** Premature ejaculation.

**Recipe** 4
**Ingredients**
cock, 1
rice wine, 500 ml

**Process** Remove the feathers and internal organs of the cock, wash it clean and cut into pieces. Put them along with a right amount of salt and vegetable oil in a pot and cook them until they are done. Add rice wine in and steam the pot in boiling water for half one hour.

**Directions** Take half of the meat twice daily.

**Indication** Premature ejaculation.

## Section 29  Emission

Emission refers to the involuntary seminal discharge that takes place often from during sexual intercourse. Specifically, nocturnal emission happens during dreams in sleep while spermatorrhea happens when the patient has no dreams or completely clear during sleep. It may be caused by prostatitis, neurasthenia, seminal vesiculitis, etc.. Seminal emission occasionally occurring in adult males, is not considered as a disease condition. Nocturnal emission in dreams is mainly due to overstrain or stress, or excessive sexual indulgence that leads to flaring up of heart fire and over consumption of kidney yin. In this case, the heart fire can not ascend to cool the heart fire, thus appearing the disharmony between the heart and kidney. The hyperactive heart fire disturbs the sperms, causing nocturnal emission in dreams. Also, functional impairment of the spleen and stomach due to over eating of sweat, greasy, fatty or pungent food can cause damp-heat accumulation in the middle jiao. The downward flowing of such a damp-heat can induce dreams and disturb the sperms, resulting in nocturnal emission. Spermatorrhea is often due to damage of the kidney after prolonged illness, over indulgence in sex or habitual masturbation. Exhausted kidney essence due to stubborn nocturnal emission causes the deficiency of kidney qi which fails to consolidate sperms. The kidney can not store sperms because the sperma gate is not firm.

### Recipe 1
**Ingredients**
Rhizoma Dioscoreae, 60 g
rice wine, 15 ml
**Process**  Grind the dried Chinese yams into fine powder. Put it along with a right amount of water in a pot. Cook it to make paste. Mix it with 15 ml of millet wine equally.
**Directions**  Take the mixture twice daily.
**Indications**  Emission, frequency of micturition due to deficiency of kidney yang.

### Recipe 2
**Ingredients**
Fructus Corni, 50 g
plain spirits, 500 ml
**Process**  Soak dogwood fruit in plain spirits and seal the container, put it in a cool, dry place for 7 days. Shake the container once daily during soaking. Filter the tincture and store it up for future administration.
**Directions**  Take 10 ml twice daily.
**Indications**  Emission, hyperhidrosis, lumbago due to deficiency of kidney qi and kidney yang.

### Recipe 3
**Ingredients**
Scorpio, 10 g
millet wine, right amount
**Process**  Bake the scorpions and then grind them into fine powder.
**Directions**  Take the powder with a right amount of millet wine to get mild perspiration.
**Indication**  Emission.

### Recipe 4
**Ingredients**
pork kidney, 1
Radix Aconiti Praeparata, 3 g
plain spirits, 10 ml
**Process**  Grind prepared aconite root into fine powder. Cut the pork kidney open and put in 3 g

of the powder. Wrap the kidney in piece of wet, clean gauze. Cook it over a slow fire until it is done.

**Directions**   Take the kidney with 10 ml of warm spirits.

**Indication**   Emission due to deficiency of kidney qi.

### Recipe 5

**Ingredients**

Semen Allii Tuberosi, 10 g

millet wine, right amount

**Process**   Decoct the Chinese chive seed in water.

**Directions**   Take the decoction with a right amount of millet wine, twice daily.

**Indication**   Emission.

### Recipe 6

**Ingredients**

Semen Cuscutae, 30 g

Fructus Schisandrae Chinensis, 30 g

plain spirits, 500 ml

**Process**   Soak Chinese magnolcavine fruit and dodder seed in plain spirits and seal the container. put it in a cool, dry place for 7 days. Shake the container once daily during soaking. Filter the tincture and store it up for future administration.

**Directions**   Take 20 ml twice daily.

**Indication**   Emission.

### Recipe 7

**Ingredients**

Semen Allii Tuberosi, 9 g

Semen Juglandis, 9 g

plain spirits, 10 ml

**Process**   Stir-fry Chinese chive seed until they become yellowish. Make decoction with the seed and walnut kernels in a right amount of water over a slow fire. Add plain spirits in boiling decoction. 5 minutes later move the pot away from the fire.

**Directions**   Take the decoction warmly twice daily.

**Indication**   Emission.

### Recipe 8

**Ingredients**

Semen Nelumbinis, 100 g

plain spirits, right amount

**Process**   Grind lotus seed into powder.

**Directions**   Take 10 g of the powder with plain spirits, twice or three times daily.

**Indication**  Emission.

**Recipe** 9
**Ingredients**
Corium Erinacei, 100 g
millet wine
**Process**  Parch hedgehog skin with its nature retained. Grind it into fine powder.
**Directions**  Take 5 g of the powder with 50 ml of warm millet wine, twice daily.
**Indication**  Emission.

## Other Proved Prescriptions

**Recipe** 1
**Ingredients**
Herba Epimedii, 200 g
plain spirits, 2000 ml
**Process**  Cut epimedium into pieces and fill a gauze bag with them. Soak the bag in plain spirits and seal the container, put it in a cool, dry place for 3 days. Shake the container once daily during soaking. Filter the tincture and store it up for future administration.
**Directions**  Take 15 ml at bed time, daily.
**Indications**  Impotency, infertility, numbness of the extremities due to deficiency of both yin and yang.

**Recipe** 2
**Ingredients**
Herba Epimedii, 62 g
Radix Rehmanniae Praeparata, 38 g
plain spirits, 1250 ml
**Process**  Cut epimedium and prepared rehmannia root into pieces and fill them in a gauze bag. Soak the bag in plain spirits and seal the container, put it in a cool, dry place for 3 days. Shake the container once daily during soaking. Filter the tincture and store it up for future administration.
**Directions**  Take 10 ml three times daily.
**Indications**  Impotency, infertility, weakness of the waist and knees, aching pain in the muscles due to deficiency of kidney yang.

**Recipe** 3

**Ingredients**

Radix Morindae Officinalis, 250 g

Herba Epimedii, 250 g

plain spirits, 1500 ml

**Process**  Cut morinda root and epimedium into pieces and fill them in a gauze bag. Soak the bag in plain spirits and seal the container, put it in a cool, dry place for 7 days. Shake the container once daily during soaking. Filter the tincture and store it up for future administration.

**Directions**  Take 20 ml twice daily.

**Indications**  Sexual hypoesthesia, neurosis, arthralgia, paralysis of the extremities, peripheral neuritis.

### Recipe 4
**Ingredients**

Cornu Cervi Pantotrichum, 15 g

Rhizoma Dioscoreae, 60 g

plain spirits, 1000 ml

**Process**  Soak pilose antler and Chinese yams in plain spirits and seal the container, put it in a cool, dry place for 7 days. Shake the container once daily during soaking. Filter the tincture and store it up for future administration.

**Directions**  Take 15 ml three times daily.

**Indication**  Sexual hypoesthesia, impotency, emission, premature ejaculation, enuresis due to deficiency of kidney yang, chronic diarrhea, aplastic anemia and other kinds of anemia.

### Recipe 5
**Ingredients**

Macrobrachium Nipponense, 12 g

Semen Cuscutae, 12 g

Semen Juglandis, 6 g

Semen Gossypii, 6 g

Cortex Eucommiae, 6 g

Radix Morindae Officinalis, 6 g

Cinnabaris, 6 g

Rhizoma Drynariae, 6 g

Fructus Lycii, 6 g

Radix Dipsaci, 6 g

Radix Achyranthis, 6 g

plain spirits, 1000 ml

**Process**  Cut the ingredients into pieces (cinnabar grinded into fine powder) and fill the ingredients except cinnabar powder in a gauze bag. Put cinnabar powder in plain spirits and stir the mixture equally. Soak the bag in the spirits and seal the container, put it in a cool, dry place for 15 days.

Shake the container once daily during soaking. Filter the tincture and store it up for future administration.

**Directions**   Take 10 to 15 ml twice daily.

**Indications**   Impotency, soreness of the waist due to deficiency of kidney yang, hypogalactia.

**Recipe** 6
**Ingredients**
Hippocampus, 2
plain spirits, 500 ml

**Process**   Soak sea horses in plain spirits and seal the container, put it in a cool, dry place for 14 days. Shake the container once daily during soaking. Filter the tincture and store it up for future administration.

**Directions**   Take 15 to 20 ml at bed time, daily.

**Indication**   Impotency, soreness of the waist and knees due to deficiency of kidney qi and essence.

**Recipe** 7
**Ingredients**
Peni et Testes Callorhini, one set
Radix Ginseng, 15 g
Rhizoma dioscoreae, 30 g
rice wine, 1000 ml

**Process**   Cut ursine seal's penis and testes into thin slices, cut ginseng and Chinese yams into pieces. Soak the ingredients in rice wine and seal the container, put it in a cool, dry place for 7 days. Shake the container once daily during soaking. Filter the tincture and store it up for future administration.

**Directions**   Take 15 ml twice daily.

**Indications**   Impotency, thinness of seminal fluid, aversion to cold, cold limbs, cold pain in the lumbar region and knees, infertility due to deficiency of kidney yang.

**Recipe** 8
**Ingredients**
Succus Lycii, 100 g
Succus Rehmanniae, 100 g
Succus Ophiopogonis, 60 g
Semen Armeniacae Amarum, 30 g
Poria, 30 g
Radix Ginseng, 20 g
plain spirits, 1500 ml

**Process**   Pound bitter apricot seed, poria and ginseng into pieces and soak them along with juices of wolfberry fruit, rehmannia root and dwarf lilyturf tuber in plain spirit and seal the container, put it in a cool, dry place for 7 days. Shake the container once daily during soaking. Filter the tincture and store it up for future administration.

**Directions**   Take 10 ml before meals, twice daily.

**Indication**   Impotency, deafness, blurring of vision, sallow face due to insufficiency of liver essence and kidney essence.

**Recipe** 9

**Ingredients**

Fructus Lycii, 80 g

Radix Rehmanniae Praeparata, 80 g

Radix Ginseng, 15 g

Poria, 20 g

Radix Polygoni Multiflori, 50 g

plain spirits, 1000 ml

**Process**   Cut the above ingredients except plain spirits into pieces and then soak them in plain spirits and seal the container, put it in a cool, dry place for 14 days. Shake the container once daily during soaking. Filter the tincture and store it up for future administration.

**Directions**   Take 10 ml twice daily.

**Indications**   Impotency, tinnitus, blurring of vision due to insufficiency of kidney essence.

**Recipe** 10

**Ingredients**

Fructus Rubi, 60 g

Semen Cuscutae, 60 g

Fructus Broussonetiae, 60 g

Fructus Rosae Laevigatae, 60 g

Fructus Lycii, 60 g

Ootheca Mantidis, 60 g

plain spirits, 2500 ml

**Process**   Cut the above ingredients except plain spirits into pieces and fill them in a gauze bag. Fasten the mouth of the bag, soak it in plain spirits and seal the container, put it in a cool, dry place for 14 days. Shake the container once daily during soaking. Filter the tincture and store it up for future administration.

**Directions**   Take 10 ml twice daily.

**Indications**   Deficiency of liver essence and kidney essence manifested by cold pain in the lumbar region and knees, lassitude and fatigue, impotency, emission, spermatorrhea, frequency of micturition, blurring of vision, leukorrhagia.

**Recipe** 11

**Ingredients**

Herba Cistanchis, 30 g

Fructus Rubi, 30 g

Fructus Psoraleae, 30 g

Fructus Mori, 23 g

Fructus Lycii, 23 g

Semen Cuscutae, 23 g

Semen Allii Tuberosi, 23 g

Fructus Broussonetiae, 23 g

Radix Morindae Officinalis, 23 g

Fructus Corni, 22 g

Radix Achyranthis, 22 g

Stamen Nelumbinis, 15 g

Fructus Cnidii, 7.5 g

Rhizoma Dioscoreae, 7.5 g

Radix Aucklandiae, 7.5 g

plain spirits, 3000 ml

**Process** Pound and grind the above ingredients except plain spirits into powder. Soak it in plain spirits in a container and cover the lid. Steam the container in boiling water for 4 hours. Then seal the container and then cover it up with earth for 2 days of time. Filter the tincture and store it up for future administration.

**Directions** Take 20 ml twice daily.

**Indications** Impotency, premature ejaculation, infertility.

**Recipe 12**

**Ingredients**

Radix Ginseng, 15 g

Radix Rehmanniae Praeparata, 15 g

Hippocampus, 10 g

Cornu Cervi Pantotrichum, 10 g

Herba Cistanchis, 20 g

plain spirits, 1000 ml

**Process** Grind ginseng and pilose antler into powder and soak it along with other ingredients in plain spirits and seal the container, put it in a cool, dry place for one month. Shake the container once daily during soaking. Filter the tincture and store it up for future administration.

**Directions** Take 10 ml twice daily.

**Indications** Sexual hypoesthesia, tinnitus, soreness of the waist and knees due to deficiency of kidney qi and yang, infertility due to deficiency of kidney yang. Contraindicated for cases with cough, fever and hypertension.

## Section 30  Simple Goiter

Simple goiter is a compensatory enlargement of the thyroid gland due to iodine deficiency. the lack of iodine in the body reduces the synthesis of thyroxin and lowers the thyroxin concentration in the blood, resulting in increased secretion of pituitary thyrotropin releasing hormone, hyperplasia and hypertrophy of the thyroid cells to lead to the enlargement of the thyroid glands. Simple goiters are more commonly seen in women and can be endemic as well as sporadic. Most goiters appear to have diffuse or nodular enlargement without pain nor abnormal change of skin color. The enlargement is soft by palpating without general symptoms. The endemic goiters have more severe enlargement of thyroid glands surrounding the neck. The enlargement may also press over nearby body organs causing dyspnea, cough, dysphagia and hoarseness of voice. Sporadic goiters, often symmetrical and lustrous, have less severe enlargement of the thyroid glands in comparison to the endemic type. The thyroid moves upward and downward with swallowing. Over a prolonged period, the goiters may turn hard or become nodular. Laboratory examinations show that the basal metabolic rate and determination of plasma protein-bound iodine appear normal.

**Recipe** 1
**Ingredients**
Rhizoma Dioscoreae, 60 g
spirits, 500 ml
**Process**  Soak the airpotato yams in the spirits and seal the container, put it in a cool, dry place for 5 days. Shake the container once daily during soaking. Filter the tincture and store it up for future administration.
**Directions**  Take 5 ml twice daily.
**Indication**  Simple goiter.

**Recipe** 2
**Ingredients**
laver, 90 g
Rhizoma Dioscoreae Bulbiferae, 60 g
spirits, 500 ml
**Process**  Soak laver and airpotato yams in spirits and seal the container, put it in a cool, dry place for 10 days. Shake the container once daily during soaking. Filter the tincture and store it up for future administration.
**Directions**  Take 15 ml twice daily.
**Indication**  Simple goiter.

**Recipe** 3
**Ingredients**
Sargassum, 500 g
Thallus Laminariae, 500 g
spirits, right amount
**Process**  Wash seaweed and kelp clean. Grind the dried seaweed and kelp into fine powder.
**Directions**  Take 20 g of the powder with a right amount of spirits twice daily.
**Indication**  Simple goiter.

**Recipe** 4
**Ingredients**
Bulbus Fritillariae Unibracteatae, 120 g
Sargassum, 120 g
Concha Ostreae, 120 g
spirits, right amount
**Process**  Grind the unibract fritillary bulbs, seaweed and oyster shell into fine powder.
**Directions**  Take 10 g of the powder with spirits twice daily.
**Indication**  Simple goiter.

## Section 31 Diabetes Mellitus

Diabetes mellitus, characterized by polydipsia, polyphagia, polyuria, emaciation and sweet urine, is the most common of the serious metabolic diseases of humans. It is a disorder of carbohydrate metabolism in which sugars in the body are not oxidized to produce energy due to lack of the pancreatic hormone insulin. The accumulation of sugar leads to its appearance in the blood (hyperglycemia), then in the urine; symptoms include thirst, loss of weight, and the excessive production of urine. The use of fats as an alternative source of energy leads to disturbances of the acid-base balance, the accumulation of ketones in the bloodstream (ketosis), and eventually to convulsions preceding diabetic coma. There appears to be an inherited tendency to diabetes; the disorder may be triggered by various factors, including physical stress. Diabetes that starts in childhood or adolescence is usually more severe than that beginning in middle or old age. Long-term complications of diabetes include thickening of the arteries, which can affect the eyes (diabetic retinopathy). According to traditional Chinese medicine, diabetes is mostly due to hyperactive heart fire and over consumption of lung yin. Retention of heat in the spleen and stomach due to improper food intake consumes the body fluid. Moreover, sexual indulgence may impair the kidney, causing the deficiency of kidney essence. These factors respectively cause the diabetes syndromes of the upper, middle and lower jiao.

**Recipe** 1
**Ingredients**
Rhizoma Polygonati, 50 g
Radix Polygoni Multiflori, 30 g
Fructus Gardeniae, 30 g
rice wine, 1000 ml

**Process**  Soak the siberian solomonseal rhizome, fleeceflower root and cape jasmine fruit in rice wine and seal the container, put it in a cool, dry place for 7 days. Shake the container once daily during soaking. Filter the tincture and store it up for future administration.

**Directions**  Take 10 ml before meals, three times daily.
**Indication**  Diabetes mellitus.

**Recipe** 2
**Ingredients**
Cipangopaludina Chinensis, 10 to 20
millet wine, 100 ml

**Process**  Wash the river snails clean, Remove the shells of the snails and mix the flesh with millet wine. Cook the mixture with a right amount of water to make soup.

**Directions**  Take the soup once daily.
**Indication**  Diabetes Mellitus.

**Recipe** 3
**Ingredients**
dried pork urinary bladdr, 10
spirits, right amount

**Process**  Wash the bladders clean and parch them with their nature retained. Then grind the parched bladder into fine powder.

**Directions**  Take 3 g of the powder with warm spirits once daily.
**Indication**  Diabetes Mellitus.

## Section 32 Hemiplegia

Hemiplegia refers to paralysis of one side of the body. Movements of the face and arm are often more severely affected than those of the leg. In this condition vascular diseases of the cerebrum and brain stem exceed all others in frequency. Cerebrovascular diseases secondary to hypertension plays an important role in the etiology. Trauma (brain contusion, epidural and subdural hemorrhage) ranks second, and other diseases such as brain tumor, brain abscess and encephalitis, demyelinative diseases, complications of meningitis, tuberculosis, and syphilis are of decreasing order of importance.

**Recipe** 1
**Ingredients**
Radix Angelicae Sinensis, 30 g
Radix Paeoniae Alba, 30 g
Radix Rehmanniae, 30 g
Radix Achyranthis Bidentatae, 30 g
Radix Gentianae Macrophyllae, 30 g
Fructus Chaenomelis, 30 g
Cortex Phellodendri, 30 g
Cortex Eucommiae, 30 g
Radix Ledebouriellae, 30 g
Radix Angelicae Dahuricae, 30 g
Pericarpium Citri Reticulatae, 30 g
Rhizoma Chuanxiong, 25 g
Rhizoma seu Radix Notopterygii, 25 g
Radix Angelicae Pubescentis, 25 g
Semen Arecae, 18 g
Cortex Cinnamomi, 10 g
Radix Glycyrrhizae Praeparata, 10 g
Lignum Pini Nodi, 15 g
plain spirits, 1600 ml

**Process** Stir-fry white peony root, phellodendron bark (with salt), eucommia bark (with ginger) until they are done. Pound and grind the above ingredients except plain spirits into powder, fill it in a bag, soak it in plain spirits in an earthenware pot, cover the lid, cook it over fire for one hour. Then take it away from the fire. After it cools, remove the bag and dregs and store the extracts up in a clean bottle for future administration.

**Directions** Take 20 ml twice daily.
**Indications** Hemiplegia, numbness of the limbs, dyskinesia.

**Recipe** 2
**Ingredients**
Semen Juglandis, 100 g
Arillus Longan, 100 g
Radix Achyranthis Bidentatae, 15 g
Cortex Eucommiae, 15 g
Herba Siegesbeckiae, 12.5 g
Rhizoma Atractylodis Macrocephalae, 12.5 g
Rhizoma Chuanxiong, 12.5 g
Radix Paeoniae Alba, 12.5 g
Poria, 12.5 g
Cortex Moutan Radicis, 12.5 g
Fructus Lycii, 25 g
Radix Polygoni Multiflori, 25 g
Radix Rehmanniae Praeparata, 25 g
Fructus Amomi, 7.5 g
Radix Linderae, 7.5 g
old wine, 1500 ml
plain spirits, 3900 ml

**Process** Pound and grind the first fourteening ingredients into powder, fill it in a gauze bag, soak it in old wine in an earthenware pot, cover the lid, cook the pot in boiling water for two hours. After it cools, add in plain spirits, seal the pot, put it in a cool, dry place for 7 days. Then remove the bag and store the extracts in a clean bottle for future administration.

**Directions** Take 20 ml twice daily.

**Indications** Hemiplegia, numbness of the limbs resulting from apoplexy due to insufficiency of liver yin and kidney essence.

**Recipe** 3
**Ingredients**
cherry, 500 g
plain spirits, 1000 ml

**Process** Wash cherries clean, soak them in plain spirits and seal the container, put it in a cool, dry place for 15 to 20 days. Stir the mixture once other day during soaking. Then filter the tincture and store it up for future administration.

**Directions** Take 30 to 50 ml twice daily.

**Indications** Hemiplegia, numbness of the limbs, arthralgia, chilblain.

**Recipe** 4
**Ingredients**
Radix Astragali, 60 g

Zaocys, 90 g

Radix Angelicae Sinensis, 40 g

Ramulus Cinnamomi, 30 g

Radix Paeoniae Alba, 25 g

plain spirits, 3000 ml

**Process**  Cut the first five ingredients into pieces, soak them in plain spirits in an earthenware pot, cover the lid, cook the pot in boiling water for one hour. After it cools, seal the pot for 7 days.

**Directions**  Take 15 ml three times daily.

**Indication**  Hemiplegia, numbness of the limbs, muscular atrophy.

**Recipe** 5

**Ingredients**

Radix Angelicae Pubescentis, 30 g

Radix Achyranthis Bidentatae, 30 g

Cortex Cinnamomi, 30 g

Radix Ledebouriellae, 30 g

Radix Aconiti Praeparata, 30 g

Fructus Cannabis, 50 g

Pericarpium Zanthoxyli, 50 g

plain spirits, 1500 ml

**Process**  Stir-fry hemp seed and bunge pricklyashpeel until they are done. Pound and grind the first seven ingredients into powder, soak it plain spirits, seal the container, put it in a cool, dry place for 3 days. Remove the dregs and store the extracts for future administration.

**Directions**  Take 5 ml before meals and at bedtime, daily.

**Indications**  Hemiplegia, arthralgia.

**Recipe** 6

**Ingredients**

Radix Angelicae Pubescentis, 20 g

Folium Photiniae, 20 g

Radix Ledebouriellae, 15 g

Herba Ephedrae, 3 g

Radix Aconiti Praeparata, 9 g

Radix Aconiti, 9 g

Cortex Cinnamomi, 9 g

Radix Achyranthis Bidentatae, 6 g

plain spirits, 800 ml

**Process**  Bake aconite root until it is done. Pound and grind the first eight ingredients into powder, soak it plain spirits, seal the container for 7 days. Remove the dregs and store the extracts up in a clean bottle for future administration.

**Directions**  Take 5 ml once daily.

**Indications**  Hemiplegia, contracture or contractive pain in the limbs, stiffness along spinal column, dyskinesia, cold pain in the abdomen.

### Recipe 7
**Ingredients**
Semen Sojae Nigrum, 125 g
Radix Salviae Miltiorrhizae, 75 g
millet wine, 1000 ml

**Process**  Pound and grind black soya beans and Dan-Shen root into powder, soak it in millet wine in a pot, cover the lid, cook it over a slow fire until one half of the wine retained. After it cools, remove the dregs and store the extracts up in a clean bottle for future administration.

**Directions**  Take 10 ml twice daily.

**Indications**  Sequelae of apoplexy such as hemiparalysis, dyskinesia.

### Recipe 8
**Ingredients**
Herba Epimedii, 50 g
Radix Morindae Officinalis, 50 g
Caulis Spatholobi, 50 g
plain spirits, 1000 ml

**Process**  Cut the first three ingredients into pieces, soak them in plain spirits, seal the container, put it in a cool, dry place for 20 days. Then remove the dregs and store the extracts up in a clean bottle for future administration.

**Directions**  Take 10 ml twice daily.

**Indications**  Hemiplegia, numbness of the limbs, arthralgia, traumatic injury.

### Recipe 9
**Ingredients**
Squama Manitis, 6 g
Radix Cynanchi Atrati, 6 g
Herba Lycopi, 6 g
plain spirits, 200 ml

**Process**  Stir-fry pangolin scales until they become yellowish, grind them into powder. Make decoction with the first three ingredients in plain spirits until 100 ml of decoction retained.

**Directions**  Take 30 ml three times daily.

**Indications**  Hemiplegia, arthralgia, podalgia.

### Recipe 10
**Ingredients**

Agkistrodon acutus, 1

Semen Oryzae Glutinosae, 1000 g

distiller's yeast, 20 g

plain spirits, 100 ml

**Process**  Soak the snake in plain spirits for one day. Then cut it open, remove the skin and bones, fill the flesh in a gauze bag for later use. Wash polished glutinous rice clean, cook it for later use. First put distiller's yeast in the bottom of an earthenware pot, put the bag on it, then place the cooked rice on the top of the bag, cover the lid and seal it carefully for 3 days (in summer) or 7 days (in winter) to make wine. Take the flesh out and dry it in the sun, grind it into powder. Filter the wine and store it up for future administration.

**Directions**  Take 0.5 g of the flesh powder with 5 ml of the wine, twice daily.

**Indication**  Hemiplegia, paralysis due to rheumatic paralysis.

**Recipe 11**
**Ingredients**
Fructus Chaenomelis, 250 g

Folium Artemisiae, 250 g

vinegar, 250 ml

rice wine, 250 ml

**Process**  Make decoction with the first two ingredients in water, add rice wine and vinegar in and stir the decoction equally.

**Directions**  First heat the diseased part with the steam of the above decoction for 20 to 30 minutes. After it cools, wash the same part with the decoction. One course consisting of 7 days.

**Indication**  Hemiplegia due to apoplexy.

## Section 33  Epilepsy

The epilepsies are a group of disorders characterized by chronic, recurrent, paroxysmal change in neurological function caused by abnormalities in the electrical activity of the brain. Each episode of neurological dysfunction is called a seizure, which is characterized by a sudden falling down in a fit, mouthful foams, eyes staring upward, convulsions and screamings as if shoutings of domesticated pigs and sheep. Epilepsy can be acquired as a result of neurological injury or a structural brain lesion and can also occur as a part of many systemic medical diseases. Epilepsy also occurs in an idiopathic form in an individual with neither a history of neurological insult nor other apparent neurological dysfunction. Isolated, nonrecurrent seizures may occur in otherwise healthy individuals for a variety of reasons, and, under these circumstances, the individual is not said to have epilepsy. According to traditional Chinese medicine, in most cases epilepsy is caused by stagnant qi circulation of the heart and liver due to fear, depression or anger, or by dampness formed in case of spleen deficiency due to improper diet. Stagnation of qi that turns into fire in a long run evaporates the dampness to form phlegm. Consequently the fire carrying phlegm to preserve into the channels and rushes up to disturb the mind, resulting in an epilepsy attack, a temporary incoordination between yin and yang.

### Recipe 1
**Ingredients**
Radix et Rhizoma Rhei, 120 g
spirits, right amount
**Process**  Soak the rhubarb in a right amount of spirits for several hours. Then decoct the rhubarb in water for 10 minutes.
**Directions**  Take the decoction once daily. One course consisting of 4 days.
**Indication**  Epilepsy.

### Recipe 2
**Ingredients**
lamb tripe
millet wine
**Process**  Bake the lamb tripe and then grind into fine powder.
**Directions**  Take 9 g of the powder with warm millet wine, once daily.
**Indication**  Epilepsy.

### Recipe 3
**Ingredients**
Stichopus Japonicus
millet wine
**Process**  Bake the sea cucumbers and then grind into fine powder.
**Directions**  Take 12 g of the powder with a right amount of warm millet wine.
**Indication**  Epilepsy.

### Recipe 4
**Ingredients**
Radix et Rhizoma Rhei, 1000 g
Radix Ledebouriellae, 500 g
spirits, 1500 ml
**Process**  Grind rhubarb and ledebouriella root into powder and then soak it in spirits and seal the container, put it in a cool, dry place for 14 days. Shake the container once daily during soaking. Filter the tincture and store it up for future administration.
**Directions**  Adults: Take 10 ml three times daily; between 10-14 years old: 5 ml three times daily; below 10 years: 5 ml twice daily.
**Indication**  Epilepsy.

**Recipe** 5
**Ingredients**
cock heart, 9
Rhizoma Bletillae, 9 g
millet wine, right amount
**Process**  Pound the cock hearts and common bletilla tuber into mash.
**Directions**  Take the mash with a right amount of millet wine twice daily.
**Indication**  Epilepsy.

## Section 34  Melancholy

Melancholy is a general term for diseases caused by emotional depression and qi stagnation. It is characterized mainly by depression, restlessness, fullness sensation in the chest, distending pain in the hypochondria, irritability or feeling of a lump in the throat. It embraces hysteria, neurosis and menopause syndrome in modern medicine. Melancholy is mostly due to emotional depression and violent rage resulting in the failure of the liver to maintain the free flow of qi, and stagnation of liver which makes upward attacks on the heart and mind. Retention of phlegm due to impairment of spleen from over thinking or poor function of spleen in transforming and transporting will turn into fire in a long run to disturb the heart and mind leading to the disturbance. Excessive anxiety or fear may also lead to melancholy because the impaired qi mechanism helps to consume nutrient blood in a hidden way.

**Recipe** 1
**Ingredients**
Arillus Longan, 250 g
plain spirits, 400 ml
**Process**  Cut longan aril into pieces and soak them in spirits and seal the container, put it in a cool, dry place for 15 to 20 days. Shake the container once daily during soaking. Filter the tincture and store it up for future administration.
**Directions**  Take the tincture 10 to 20 ml twice daily.
**Indication**  Neurosis.

**Recipe** 2
**Ingredients**
Semen Persicae, 10 g
white sugar, 20 g
millet wine, 50 ml

**Process**  Pound peach kernels and white sugar into mash. Decoct the mash with millet wine over a slow fire for 10 minutes.

**Directions**  Take the decoction twice daily.

**Indication**  Neurosis.

### Recipe 3
**Ingredients**

Ganoderma Lucidum, 30 g

plain spirits, 500 ml

**Process**  Cut lucid ganoderma into pieces and soak them in 500 ml of spirits and seal the container, put it in a cool, dry place for 15 days. Shake the container three times daily during soaking. Filter the tincture and store it up for future administration.

**Directions**  Take 10 ml once or twice daily.

**Indication**  Neurosis.

### Recipe 4
**Ingredients**

Fructus Ligustri Lucidi, 250 g

rice wine, 500 ml

**Process**  Soak the glossy privet fruit in rice wine and seal the container, put it in a cool, dry place for one month. Shake the container once daily during soaking. Filter the extracts and store it up for future administration.

**Directions**  Take a right amount of extracts once or twice daily.

**Indication**  Neurosis.

### Recipe 5
**Ingredients**

Radix Ginseng, 50 g

plain spirits, 500 ml

**Process**  Pound ginseng into pieces and then soak them in spirits and seal the container, put it in a cool, dry place for 15 days. Shake the container once daily during soaking. Filter the tincture and store it up for future administration. daily.

**Directions**  Take 10 ml before supper, daily.

**Indication**  Neurosis.

### Recipe 6
**Ingredients**

Ganoderma Lucidum, 30 g

Radix Salviae Miltiorrhizae, 5 g

Radix Notoginseng, 5 g

spirits, 500 ml

**Process**   Soak lucid ganoderma, Dan-Shen root and notoginseng in spirits and seal the container, put it in a cool, dry place for 15 days. Shake the container once daily during soaking. Filter the tincture and store it up for future administration.

**Directions**   Take 10 ml once daily.

**Indications**   Neurosis, insomnia.

### Recipe 7
**Ingredients**

Fructus Lycii, 500 g

spirits, 2000 ml

**Process**   Pound wolfberry fruit into powder. Soak it in spirits and seal the container, put it in a cool, dry place for 15 days. Shake the container once daily during soaking. Filter the tincture and store it up for future administration.

**Directions**   Take 5 ml three times daily.

**Indication**   Neurosis.

### Recipe 8
**Ingredients**

Rhizoma Polygonati, 50 g

Radix Polygoni Multiflori, 30 g

Fructus Lycii, 30 g

rice wine, 1000 ml

**Process**   Soak siberian Solomonseal rhizome, fleeceflower root and wolfberry fruit in rice wine and seal the container, put it in a cool, dry place for 7 days. Shake the container once daily during soaking. Filter the extracts and store it up for future administration.

**Directions**   Take 10 ml before meals, three times daily.

**Indication**   Neurosis.

### Recipe 9
**Ingredients**

pork spinal cord, one set

millet wine, 500 ml

**Process**   Cut the spinal cord into pieces. Put them in an earthenware pot and add millet wine in. Cook them over a slow fire until they are done.

**Directions**   Take half of them twice daily.

**Indication**   Neurosis.

### Recipe 10
**Ingredients**

Radix Cyperi, 60 g

white spirits, 250 ml

**Process**  Cut nutgrass flatsedge root into pieces and soak them in 250 ml of water and 250 ml of white spirits. Seal the container, put it in a cool, dry place for 3 to 5 days. Shake the container once daily during soaking. Filter the tincture and store it up for future administration.

**Directions**  Take 20 ml three times daily.

**Indication**  Depression.

## Section 35  Amnesia

Amnesia refers to total or partial loss of memory following physical injury, disease, drugs, or psychological trauma. An amnesic syndrome can be seen in various kinds of diseases. Amnesic syndrome of sudden onset (usually with gradual but incomplete recovery) is caused by A) bilateral hippocampal infarction due to atherosclerotic-thrombotic or embolic occlusion of the posterior cerebral arteries or their inferior temporal branches; B) Trauma to the diencephalic or inferomedial temporal regions; C) spontaneous subarachnoid hemorrhage; D) carbon monoxide poisoning and other hypoxic states (rare). Amnesia of sudden onset and brief duration with full recovery is due to A) temporal lobe seizures; B) postconcussive states; C) "transient global amnesia". Amnesic syndrome of subacute onset with varying degrees of recovery (usually leaving permanent residue) is due to A) Wernicke-Korsakoff disease; B) inclusion body (herpes simplex) encephalitis; C) tuberculous and other forms of meningitis characterized by a granulomatous exudate at the base of the brain. Slowly progressive amnesic states is caused by A) tumors involving the walls of the third ventricle and temporal lobes; B) alzheimer's diseases and other degenerative disorders (early stage only). In traditional Chinese medicine, Amnesia, also known as poor memory, refers to a condition characterized by hypomnesis and forgetfulness. Amnesia discussed in traditional Chinese medicine is seen in patients suffering from neurasthenia, cerebral arteriosclerosis in modern medicine. Amnesia involves a perplexing etiology, it is mostly caused by impairment of the heart and spleen as well as deficiency of heart and spleen due to overthinking. Kidney yin deficiency due to excessive sexual indulgence may create a disharmony between the heart and kidney, resulting in poor memory. Besides, poor nourishment of the brain due to kidney deficiency in the aged and deficiency of heart qi, or obstruction of the heart by phlegm-fluid retention and blood stasis may also cause poor memory.

**Recipe 1**

**Ingredients**

Radix Ophiopogonis, 30 g

Semen Biotae, 15 g

Poria, 15 g

Radix Rehmanniae, 22 g

Arillus Longan, 15 g

spirit, 2500 ml

**Process**　Cut dwarf lilyturf tuber, arborvitae seed, poria, Chinese angelica, longan aril and rehmannia root into pieces and fill them in a gauze bag. Soak it in spirit and seal the container, put it in a cool, dry place. 7 days later remove the dregs and filter the tincture, store it up for future administration.

**Directions**　Take 10-15 ml twice daily.

**Indications**　Amnesia due to deficiency of yin and blood manifested by amnesia accompanied by restlessness, palpitation, insomnia, listlessness.

**Recipe** 2

**Ingredients**

Arillus Longan, 250 g

sweet-scented osmanthus, 60 g

white sugar, 120 g

spirit, 2500 g

**Process**　Soak longan aril, sweet-scented osman thus and white sugar in spirit and seal the container, put it in a cool, dry place for a long time. Shake the container once daily during soaking. Filter the tincture and store it up for future administration.

**Directions**　Take 15-20 ml twice daily.

**Indications**　Amnesia, neurosis, general weakness, insomnia, palpitation. Contraindicated for cases with diabetes.

**Recipe** 3

**Ingredients**

Poria, 60 g

spirit, 500 ml

**Process**　Cut poria into small pieces. Soak them in spirit and seal the container, put it in a cool, dry place for 7 days. Shake the container once daily during soaking. Filter the tincture and store it up for future administration.

**Directions**　Take 10-15 ml twice daily.

**Indications**　Deficiency of the spleen marked by amnesia, general lassitude, flaccidity syndrome, palpitation and insomnia.

**Recipe** 4

**Ingredients**

Fructus Lycii, 18 g

Poria, 18 g

Radix Rehmanniae, 18 g

Radix Rehmanniae Praeparata, 18 g

Fructus Corni, 18 g

Radix Achyranthis Bidentatae, 18 g

Radix Polygalae, 18 g

Cortex Acanthopanacis Radicis, 18 g

Rhizoma Acori Graminei, 18 g

Cortex Lycii Radicis, 18 g

spirit, 1500 ml

**Process**  Cut the drugs into pieces and then fill in a gauze bag. Soak the bag in spirit and seal the container, put it in a cool, dry place for 14 days. Shake the container once daily during soaking. Filter the tincture and store it up for future administration.

**Directions**  Take 20 ml once daily.

**Indication**  Amnesia due to deficiency of heart blood and kidney essence.

**Note:**  Containers made of either iron or copper prohibited.

**Recipe 5**
**Ingredients**

Semen Persicae, 100 g

Cinnabaris, 10 g

old wine, 500 ml

**Process**  Bake peach kernel over a slow fire until it becomes brown. Grind cinnabar into fine powder. Soak peach kernels in old wine and cover the lid of the container. Heat the container over fire until the decoction boils. Add cinnabar in when the decoction cools, stir the mixture equally for future administration.

**Directions**  Take 10 to 15 ml twice daily.

**Indications**  Amnesia, palpitation, pale complexion, pain due to spasm of the muscles.

## Section 36  Insomnia

Insomnia is a condition that makes the patient unable to acquire normal hours of sleep. It is usually accompanied by dizziness, headache, palpitation and poor memory. Insomnia presents different manifestations in the clinic. In the mild cases, there may be difficulty in falling into sleep, dream disturbed sleep that often wakes up the patient with frightening or makes one unable to fall into sleep again. In severe cases, there can often be no sleep for the whole night. Insomnia can be due to various causative factors. Impairment of the heart and spleen by over thinking or overstrain causes insufficiency of qi and blood which fail to nourish the heart and calm the mind. Impairment of the kidney due to sexual indulgence can cause kidney yin deficiency and hyperactive fire that leads to disharmony between the spleen and stomach due to improper diet leads to excessive accumulation of dampness and phlegm. And stagnant phlegm produces fire which flares up to disturb the heart and mind. Stagnation of liver qi turning into fire due to emotional disturbance can cause flaring up of liver fire to disturb the heart and mind, resulting in insomnia.

**Recipe** 1
**Ingredients**
Cordyceps, 30 g
spirit, 500 ml
**Process**  Soak Chinese caterpillar fungus in 500 ml of spirits, seal the container and put it in a cool, dry place for 7 days. Shake the container once daily during soaking. Filter the tincture and store it up for future administration.
**Directions**  Take 10-20 ml twice to three times daily.
**Indication**  Insomnia due to yin deficiency.

**Recipe** 2
**Ingredients**
Poria, 30 g
Semen Biotae, 30 g
Radix Angelicae Sinensis, 30 g
Radix Rehmanniae, 45 g
Ziziphi Spinosae, 15 g
Radix Ophiopogonis, 60 g
Arillus Longan, 60 g
spirit, 3000 ml
**Process**  Fill poria, arborvitae seed, Chinese angelica, dried rehmannia root, spine date seed, dwarf lilyturf tuber and longan aril in a gauze bag and soak it in spirits. Seal the container, put it in a cool, dry place for 15 days. Shake the container once daily during soaking. Filter the tincture and store it up for future administration.
**Directions**  Take 30 ml of the tincture twice daily.
**Indications**  Insomnia due to deficiency of heart blood and spleen qi manifested by palpitation, general lassitude, pale complexion, restlessness, insomnia and dreaminess.

**Recipe** 3
**Ingredients**
Arillus Longan, 250 g
spirit, 1500 ml
**Process**  Soak longan aril in 1500 ml of spirit and seal the container, put it in a cool, dry place for one month. Shake the container once daily during soaking. Filter the tincture and store it up for future administration.

**Directions**  Take 15 to 25 ml twice daily.

**Indications**  Insomnia accompanied with consumption, palpitation, amnesia, indigestion, anorexia.

### Recipe 4
**Ingredients**

Arillus Longan, 125 g

Caulis Spatholobi, 125 g

Radix Polygoni Multiflori, 125 g

spirit, 1500 ml

**Process**  Cut fleece-flower root and suberect spatholobus stem into pieces. Soak them along with longan aril in spirit and seal the container, put it in a cool, dry place for 10 days. Remove the dregs and store the tincture for later use.

**Directions**  Take 20 ml twice daily.

**Indications**  Insomnia accompanied by anemia, weight loss, neurosis, amnesia.

### Recipe 5
**Ingredients**

Radix Salviae Miltiorrhizae, 30 g

spirit, 1000 ml

**Process**  Soak Dan-Shen root in 1000 ml of spirit and seal the container, put it in a cool, dry place for 3 to 5 days. Shake the container once daily during soaking. Filter the tincture and store it up for future administration.

**Directions**  Take 10 ml before sleep.

**Indication**  Insomnia.

### Recipe 6
**Ingredients**

Ganoderma Lucidum, 100 g

rice wine, 1000 ml

**Process**  Cut lucid ganoderma into pieces. Soak them in rice wine and seal the container, put it in a cool, dry place for 7 days. Shake the container once daily during soaking. Filter the tincture and store it up for future administration.

**Directions**  Take 10 ml of the tincture twice daily.

**Indication**  Insomnia and amnesia.

### Recipe 7
**Ingredients**

Fructus Schisandrae Chinensis, 50 g

spirit, 500 ml

**Process**  Soak Chinese magnolcavine fruit in spirit and seal the container, put it in a cool, dry place for 15 days. Shake the container once daily during soaking. Filter the tincture and store it up for future administration.

**Directions**  Take 3 ml after meals three times daily

**Indication**  Insomnia due to neurosis.

### Recipe 8
**Ingredients**
walnut kernel, 10 g
white sugar, 20 g
millet wine, 50 ml

**Process**  Pound walnut kernel along with white sugar into paste. Add in 500 ml of millet wine and decoct the mixture over a slow fire for 15 minutes.

**Directions**  Take all the decoction twice daily.

**Indication**  Insomnia due to neurosis.

### Recipe 9
**Ingredients**
Semen Cuscutae, 30 g
Fructus Schisandrae Chinensis, 30 g
spirit, 500 ml

**Process**  Soak Chinese magnolcavine fruit and pepperweed seed in 500 ml of spirit and seal the container, put it in a cool, dry place for 7 days. Shake the container once daily during soaking. Filter the tincture and store it up for future administration.

**Directions**  Take 5 ml of the tincture three times daily.

**Indication**  Insomnia due to neurosis.

### Recipe 10
**Ingredients**
Radix Ginseng, 50 g
spirit, 500 ml

**Process**  Pound ginseng into pieces and fill them in a bottle. Add 500 ml of spirit in and seal the bottle for 15 days. Shake the bottle once daily.

**Directions**  Take 10 ml of the tincture before supper.

**Indication**  Insomnia due to deficiency of spleen qi.

### Recipe 11
**Ingredients**
Flos Chrysanthemi, 30 g
Radix Rehmanniae, 10 g

Radix Angelicae Sinensis, 10 g

Fructus Lycii, 20 g

spirit, 500 ml

**Process**  Soak chrysanthemum flowers, rehmannia root, Chinese angelica and wolfberry fruit in spirit and seal the container, put it in a cool, dry place for 7 days. Shake the container once daily during soaking. Filter the tincture and store it up for future administration.

**Directions**  Take 10 ml three times daily.

**Indications**  Dreaminess or insomnia.

## Section 37  Parotitis

Parotitis, also known as mumps, is an acute infectious disease caused by invasion of exogenous pathogenic wind-heat. Clinically, it is characterized by fever, pain and swelling in the parotid region. It occurs all year round with higher incidence in children between five to nine years old, particularly in spring. The prognosis of this disease is often favorable. The onset is mainly due to invasion of exogenous pathogenic wind-heat into the Shaoyang Channels. The deranged qi mechanism of the Shaoyang Channels with impaired circulation of qi and blood causes pain and swelling in the parotid region, fever with aversion to cold. The Shaoyang channels and the Jueyin Channels are internally-externally related channels. The Liver Meridian of Foot-Jueyin curves around the pubic region. Extreme heat descending along this particular channel may result in swelling and pain in the testis. However, there will be high fever, convulsion and coma provided that the pathogenic heat runs into the pericardium along the Pericardium Meridian of Hand-Jueyin to disturb the mind.

Note: The dosage of every prescription is used in adulthood.

**Recipe 1**

**Ingredients**

Fructus Luffae, 1

millet wine, right amount

**Process**  Cut luffa into pieces and then stir-fry them until they become yellowish. Grind the pieces into fine powder.

**Directions**  Take 9 g of the powder three times daily.

**Indication**  Parotitis.

**Recipe 2**

**Ingredients**

Indigo Naturalis, 9 g

egg, 1

spirits, right amount

**Process**   Mix egg white with indigo equally.
**Directions**   Take the mixture with warm spirits of a right amount, once daily.
**Indication**   Parotitis.

## Recipe 3
**Ingredients**
Semen Sinapis Albae, 150 g
plain spirits, 250 ml
**Process**   Fill a gauze bag with white mustard seed and fasten the mouth of the bag. Put the bag along with spirits in an earthenware pot. Decoct the ingredients over fire until it boils.
**Directions**   Apply the hot bag on the diseased region, twice to four times daily; take 5 ml of the decoction twice or three times daily.
**Indication**   Parotitis. Contraindicated for cases with allergic skin.

## Recipe 4
**Ingredients**
Radix Sophorae Subprostratae, 15 g
spirits, right amount
water, right amount
**Process**   Wash subprostrate sophora root clean and pound into mash. Make decoction with the mash and right amount of spirits and water to get thick decoction.
**Directions**   Apply the decoction on the diseased area twice to three times daily.
**Indication**   Parotitis.

## Recipe 5
**Ingredients**
Pericarpium Zanthoxyli, 50 grains
Cacumen Platycladi Orientalis, 15 g
spirits, 500 ml
**Process**   Grind bunge pricklyash peel into fine powder and pound oriental arborvitae leafy twigs into mash. Soak the powder and mash in spirits and seal the container, put it in a cool, dry place for 15 days. Shake the container once daily during soaking. Filter the tincture and store it up for future administration.
**Directions**   Take 5 to 10 ml every morning.
**Indication**   Parotitis.

## Section 38  Malaria

Malaria is an infectious disease characterized by shivering chills and strong fever at regular intervals. This condition can be divided into quotidian malaria, tertian malaria and quartan malaria according to the interval between every two attacks. There may be some palpable mass in the hypochondriac region in the chronic case. And this is medically called malaria with splenomegaly. Malaria is seen more common in summer and autumn, and may also sporadically occur in other seasons. It is mainly caused by the invasion of pestilential factor and that of exogenous pathogenic heat, wind, cold and dampness dormant in the semi-exterior and semi-interior and wandering between the nutrient and defensive systems. Chills appear if such factors run into the nutrient system, and heat occurs if they outwardly disturb the defensive system. The imbalance between nutrient and defensive systems and the struggle between the anti-pathogenic qi and pathogenic qi develop malaria.

**Recipe** 1
**Ingredients**
Mel, 30 g
spirits, 3 drops
**Process**  Mix the honey and spirits well.
**Directions**  Take the honey and spirits with warm water one hour before the attack of malaria.
**Indication**  Malaria.

**Recipe** 2
**Ingredients**
Radix Dichroae, 3 g
Fructus Tsaoko, 3 g
Flos Caryophylli, 3 g
old spirits, 10 ml
**Process**  Make decoction with the above ingredients (soak dichroa root, tsaoko cardamon and cloves before decocting) until it has been brought to boils of several times.
**Directions**  Inhale the medicated steam one hour before the attack of malaria.
**Indication**  Malaria.

**Recipe** 3
**Ingredients**
Pericarpium Zanthoxyli, 20 grains
rice wine, 60 ml
**Process**  Pound the bunge pricklyash peel into powder. Make decoction with the powder along with right amount of water.

**Directions**  Take the decoction with warm millet wine.
**Indication**  Malaria marked by severe aversion to cold and mild fever.

**Recipe** 4
**Ingredients**
Bulbus Allii, 20 g
rice wine, right amount
**Process**  Pound the garlic into mash.
**Directions**  Take the mash with warm rice wine one hour before the attack of malaria.
**Indication**  Malaria.

**Recipe** 5
**Ingredients**
Os Sepiella seu Sepiae, 3 g
spirits, 10 ml
**Process**  Grind the cuttle-bone into powder.
**Directions**  Take the powder with spirits one hour before the attack of malaria.
**Indication**  Malaria.

**Recipe** 6
**Ingredients**
Plastrum Testudinis, 30 g
spirits, right amount
**Process**  Parch tortoise plastron with its nature retained. Grind the parched plastron into fine powder.
**Directions**  Take 3 g of the powder with 5 to 10 ml of spirits.
**Indication**  Chronic malaria.

**Recipe** 7
**Ingredients**
egg, 1
spirits, 20 ml
**Process**  Mix the egg white with spirits equally.
**Directions**  Take the mixture twice to three times one week for prevention of malaria. Double the dosage for treatment.
**Indication**  Malaria.

**Recipe** 8
**Ingredients**
Herba Artemisiae, 1000 g

Semen Oryzae Glutinosae, 500 g

distiller's yeast, right amount

**Process** Wash sweet wormwood clean and pound into mash to extract juice. Cook the polished glutinous rice along with the juice until it is done. after it cools, mix the rice with a right amount of distiller's yeast equally to make wine.

**Directions** Take right amount of such rice wine one hour before the attack of malaria.

**Indication** Malaria.

## Section 39  Dysentery

Dysentery is an intestinal epidemic disease that occurs more in the summer time. It is characterized by abdominal pain, tenesmus and frequent bowel motions containing blood and mucous. Clinically, it is divided into damp-heat dysentery, damp-cold dysentery, fasting dysentery and chronic recurrent dysentery. This condition in most cases is caused by impairment of the stomach and intestine due to improper intake of raw, cold or unclean food, or due to invasion of damp-heat in summer. If the excessive damp-heat turns into fire steaming the blood and impairing the intestinal collaterals, there will be bloody stools impairing the intestinal collaterals, there will be bloody stools with more blood and less pus, known as the damp-heat type of dysentery. If excessive cold-damp affects and retains in the intestines, the dysentery will involve with white mucous or with more pus but less white mucous, known as the cold-damp type dysentery. In case of pathogenic heat invading the stomach, such symptoms and signs as nausea, vomiting and complete loss of appetite will occur, known as the fasting dysentery. If the above mentioned dysenteries have undergone a long course, resulting in qi deficiency in the middle jiao and weakness of body resistance against pathogenic factor invading, chronic recurrent dysentery occurs.

**Recipe 1**

**Ingredients**

eggs of tortoise

spirits.

**Process** Cook the eggs in boiling water until they are done.

**Directions** Take the eggs with a right amount of spirits.

**Indication** Dysentery.

**Recipe 2**

**Ingredients**

red bayberry

old spirits

**Process** Soak the red bayberries in old spirits, seal the container and put it in a cool, dry place for three days.

**Directions** Take one or two bayberries twice daily.
**Indication** Dysentery.

**Recipe** 3
**Ingredients**
rose

millet wine

**Process** Bake the flowers and then grind the dried flowers into fine powder.
**Directions** Take 2 g of the powder with warm millet wine, twice to three times daily.
**Indication** Dysentery.

**Recipe** 4
**Ingredients**
Folium Persicae, 15 g

egg, 1

spirit, right amount

**Process** Decoct the peach leaves and egg with spirits until the the egg is done and in the mean time all the spirits changes into vapor.
**Directions** Take one egg three times daily.
**Indication** Dysentery.

**Recipe** 5
**Ingredients**
crucian carp, 1

brown sugar, right amount

old spirits, right amount

**Process** Remove the internal organs of the fish and parch it with its nature retained. Grind the parched fish into fine powder and mix it with brown sugar equally.
**Directions** Take 9 g of the mixture once daily.
**Indications** Chronic dysentery, chronic dysentery with frequent relapse.

**Recipe** 6
**Ingredients**
eel

brown sugar

millet wine

**Process** Remove the internal organs of the eels and parch them with their nature retained. Grind the parched eels into fine powder. Mix it with a right amount of brown sugar equally.
**Directions** Take 9 g of the mixture with right amount of warm millet wine.

**Indication** Dysentery.

**Recipe 7**
**Ingredients**
Fructus Crataegi, 60 g
brown sugar, 10 g
spirits, 30 ml

**Process** Bake the hawthorn fruit over a slow fire until their outer parts become charred. After they cool, add 30 ml of spirits in and mix them. Then stir-fry the fruit over fire until all the spirits changes into vapor. Add 200 ml in and decoct the fruit for 15 minutes. Remove the dregs and add 10 g of brown sugar in the decoction and mix it equally, then heat it over fire until it boils.
**Directions** Take the decoction warmly, once daily.
**Indication** Dysentery.

**Recipe 8**
**Ingredients**
pig bone, 90 g
spirits, right amount

**Process** Parch the bones with the nature retained. Grind the parched bones into powder.
**Directions** Take 9 g of the powder with right amount of warm spirits, once daily.
**Indication** Dysentery.

**Recipe 9**
**Ingredients**
cucumber
brown sugar, 9 g
white sugar, 9 g
spirits

**Process** Soak the cucumber in a right amount of spirits and seal the container, put it in a cool, dry place for 21 days. Cut the cucumber into lengths the length of 3 cm long.
**Directions** Take one length of cucumber along with sugar once daily.
**Indication** Dysentery.

**Recipe 10**
**Ingredients**
Radix Ginseng, 20 g
Radix Aconiti Praeparata, 20 g
Radix et Rhizoma Rhei, 50 g
Rhizoma Zingiberis, 30 g
Radix Glycyrrhizae, 20 g

millet wine, 1000 ml

**Process**  Grind ginseng, prepared aconite root, rhubarb, dried ginger and liquorice into powder. Fill a gauze bag with the powder. Soak the bag with millet wine and seal the container, put it in a cool, dry place for two months. Shake the container once daily during soaking. Filter the tincture and store it up for future administration.

**Directions**  Take 5 ml once to twice daily. One course consisting of three or seven days.

**Indication**  Chronic dysentery of cold type.

# Chapter Two Surgical Diseases

## Section 1 Furuncle, Carbuncle and Cellulitis

Furuncle refers to a tender inflamed area of the skin containing pus. the infection is usually caused by the bacterium Staphylococcus aureus entering through a hair follicle or a break in the skin, and local injury or lowered constitutional resistance may encourage the development of boils. Boils usually heal when the pus is released or with antibiotic treatment, though occasionally they may cause more widespread infection. Carbuncle refers to a collection of boils with multiple drainage channels. The infection normally results in an extensive slough of skin. While cellulitis refers to inflammation of the connective tissue between adjacent tissues and organs. This is commonly due to bacterial infection and usually requires antibiotic treatment to prevent its spread to the bloodstream.

**Recipe 1**
**Ingredients**
Flos Lonicerae, 20 g
Herba Taraxaci, 15 g
Flos Chrysanthemi Indici, 15 g
Herba Violae, 15 g
Radix Semiaquilegiae, 15 g
millet wine, right amount
**Process** Make decoction with the above ingredients except milletwine in water.
**Directions** Take one half of the decoction with a right amount of warm millet wine, twice daily. One course consists of 3 days.
**Indication** Nail-like boil.

**Recipe 2**
**Ingredients**
Flos Sophorae, 60 g
Semen Juglandis, 60 g
plain spirits, 120 ml
**Process** Make decoction with sophora flowers and walnut kernels in plain spirits until 60 ml of decoction retained.
**Directions** Take one half of the decoction, twice daily.
**Indication** Nail-like boil.

**Recipe** 3
**Ingredients**
Fructus Litchi, 5
Thallus Laminariae, 15 g
millet wine, 20 ml
**Process**  Make decoction with litchis and kelp along with millet wine in 100 ml of water until 60 ml of decoction retained.
**Directions**  Take one half of the decoction twice daily.
**Indication**  Nail-like boil.

**Recipe** 4
**Ingredients**
Calyx Cucurbitae, 25 g
millet wine, right amount
vinegar, right amount
**Process**  Parch pumpkin calyces with their nature retained. Grind the parched calyces into fine powder.
**Directions**  Take 2.5 g of the powder with a right amount of warm millet wine, twice daily. Also applied on affected part with a right amount of vinegar.
**Indicatins**  Furuncle, nail-like boil.

**Recipe** 5
**Ingredients**
Radix Angelicae Sinensis, 15 g
Radix Angelicae Dahuricae, 12 g
Spica Prunellae, 9 g
Rhizoma Chuanxiong, 12 g
Radix Achyranthis Bidentatae, 15 g
plain spirits, 200 ml
water, 200 ml
**Process**  Mix plain spirits and water equally in an earth enware pot. Put the other ingredients in the pot and make decoction with them.
**Directions**  Take one half of the decoction twice daily.
**Indication**  Skin and external diseases including carbuncle, furuncle, multiple abscess, ulcer, etc..

**Recipe** 6
**Ingredients**
crab, 2
millet wine, 100 ml

**Process**  Wash the crabs clean and pound them into mash. Soak the mash in millet wine for one hour. Filter the tincture and put the extracts in a bowl.
**Directions**  Take the extracts warmly.
**Indication**  Carbuncle, phlegmon, furuncle, nail-like boil.

### Recipe 7
**Ingredients**
Radix Lobeliae Radicantis, 10 g
distiller's yeast, 5 g
**Process**  Wash the root of radical lobelia clean and pound it into mash. Mix it with distiller's yeast equally and pound the mixture.
**Directions**  Apply the mixture on affected part, twice or three times daily. 3 days consisted of one course.
**Indication**  Pustule of the finger tip.

### Recipe 8
**Ingredients**
Folium Chrysanthemi Indici
vinegar
distiller's yeast
**Process**  Wash the leaves clean and pound them into mash. Mix it with vinegar and distiller's yeast and pound again.
**Directions**  Apply the mixture on affected part.
**Indication**  Pustule of the finger tip.

### Recipe 9
**Ingredients**
Cera Flava, 30 g
Radix Angelicae Dahuricae, 45 g
distiller's yeast, right amount
**Process**  Parch beeswax with its nature retained. Grind it along with dahurian angelica root into fine powder. Mix the powder with distiller's yeast equally.
**Directions**  Apply on affected part, twice daily. One course consisting of 3 days.
**Indication**  Lumbodorsal carbuncle.

### Recipe 10
**Ingredients**
Cacumen Platycladi Orientalis, 30 g
Alumen, 3 g
plain spirits, 30 ml

**Process**　　Grind alum into fine powder and dissolve it in spirits. Pound oriental arborvitae leafytwigs into mash. Put the mash in the solution of alum and mix equally.

**Directions**　　Apply the mixture on affected part, once daily.

**Indicatins**　　Carbuncle, deep abscess.

**Recipe** 11
**Ingredients**
Colophonium, 10 g
plain spirits, right amount

**Process**　　Grind colophony into fine powder and mix it with plain spirits. Put the mixture in cup and cover the lid. Heat the mixture in boiling water until it changes into liquid thoroughly.

**Directions**　　Spread liquid colophony over the affected part. Cover the part with a piece of wax paper.

**Indication**　　Furuncle, carbuncle, folliculitis.

## Section 2　　Lymphadenitis

Lymphadenitis refers to inflammation of lymph nodes, which become swollen, painful, and tender. Some cases may be chronic but most are acute and localized adjacent to an area of infection. The most commonly affected lymph nodes are those in the neck, in association with tonsillitis. The lymph nodes help to contain and combat the infection. Occasionally generalized lymphadenitis occurs as a result of virus infections.

**Recipe**
**Ingredients**
Folium Persicae, 10 g
millet wine, right amount

**Process**　　Pound the leaves into mash and stir-fry it with its nature retained. Mix it with millet wine equally.

**Directions**　　Apply the mixture on affected part.

**Indication**　　Lymphadenitis.

# Section 3  Lymphoid Tuberculosis

Lymphoid tuberculosis, also known as scrofula, refers to masses of irregular sizes without redness, feverish sensation, nor obvious pain in the posterior area of the ear, neck or nape. There can be one or several masses in line, leading to abscesses. This condition is usually due to phlegm-fire accumulating in the neck by the action of pathogenic fire consuming the body fluid, resulting from emotional upsets and prolonged stagnation of liver qi, or due to ascending of qi with phlegm located in the neck resulting from dominant nation of liver yang and consumption of body fluid, which is caused by deficiency of lung yin and kidney yin. The prolonged accumulation of phlegm and qi may turn into excessive heat leading to erosion and discharge of pus. It is slow to heal and may require prolonged treatment.

### Recipe 1
**Ingredients**
Cortex Lycii Radicis, 10 g
millet wine, 100 ml
**Process**  Soak wolfberry bark in millet wine and seal the container for 7 days. Filter the tincture and store the extracts up in a clean bottle for future administration.
**Directions**  Take 10 ml before meals three times daily.
**Indication**  Lymphoid tuberculosis.

### Recipe 2
**Ingredients**
Semen gossypii, 300 g
white sugar, right amount
plain spirits, right amount
**Process**  Stir-fry cotton seed to dry, then stir with plain spirits, parch them until they become brown. Pound and grind the parched seed into fine powder and mix it with white sugar. Store the mixture up in a clean bottle for future administration.
**Directions**  Take 10 g three times daily. One course consisting of one months.
**Indication**  Lymphoid tuberculosis.

### Recipe 3
**Ingredients**
Fructus Litchi, 50 g
Sargassum, 15 g
Thallus Laminariae, 15 g

millet wine, 20 ml
**Process**   Make decoction with the above ingredients in water.
**Directions**   Take one half of the decoction twice daily.
**Indication**   Lymphoid tuberculosis.

**Recipe** 4
**Ingredients**
pod of sword bean, 30 g
egg, 1
plain spirits, 50 ml
**Process**   Make decoction with the above ingredients in water.
**Directions**   Take one half of the decoction twice daily.
**Indication**   Lymphoid tuberculosis.

**Recipe** 5
**Ingredients**
Thallus Laminariae, 500 g
plain spirits, 1000 ml
**Process**   Wash the kelp clean and cut into pieces. Soak them in 1000 ml of plain spirits and seal the container for 20 days. Filter the mixture and store the extracts up in a clean bottle for future administration.
**Directions**   Take 10 ml twice daily.
**Indication**   Lymphoid tuberculosis.

## Section 4   Osseous Tuberculosis

Hematogenous spread of tuberculosis to the long bones and vertebrae is most common when infection occurs in childhood, because of the high pressure of oxygen associated with the vascularity at the epiphyseal plates during active bone growth. It usually occurs within three years of infection, but dormant lesions may be reactivated by trauma years later. Infection begins in the ends of the long bones but becomes obvious when it involves the adjacent joint: hip, knee, elbow, or wrist. Tenosynovitis is most common at the wrist.

**Recipe** 1
**Ingredients**
Radix Aconiti Kusnezoffii, 50 g
Radix Paeoniae Rubra, 20 g
Cortex Cinnamomi, 25 g

plain spirits, right amount

**Process**   Grind wild aconite root, red peony root and cassia bark into fine powder.

**Directions**   Apply a right amount of powder on affected part with plain spirits.

**Indication**   Primary osseous tuberculosis.

**Recipe** 2

**Ingredients**

Radix Aconiti Praeparata, 12 g

argyi wool, 30 g

plain spirits

**Process**   Pound prepared aconite root and argyi wool into mash.

**Directions**   Apply the mash on affected part with a right amount of plain spirits, then give moxibustion with moxa sticks for 10 minutes, twice daily.

**Indication**   Osseous tuberculosis.

## Section 5   Mastitis

Mastitis, or breast abscess, a kind of acute purulent infection of the breast, is mostly seen during lactation period, especially in primiparae. It is mostly caused by emotional disturbance and stagnation of liver qi that leads to dysfunction of liver in maintaining free flow of qi and stagnant lactation, or by improper diet such as over indulgence of greasy food that leads to dysfunction of spleen qi in ascending and descending qi of stomach as well as heat retention in the stomach. However, broken nipple with exogenous invasion that encounters the internal heat can also cause stagnant lactation. Stagnant lactation in a long run will also turn into heat with excessive heat retention in the local area that develops into mastitis.

**Recipe** 1

**Ingredients**

Semen Citri Reticulatae, 15 g

millet wine, right amount

**Process**   Make decoction with tangerine seed in millet wine. Filter the decoction and store the extracts up in a bowl.

**Directions**   Take one half of the decoction warmly, twice daily.

**Indication**   Primary mastitis.

**Recipe** 2

**Ingredients**

Radix Rhapontici seu Echinopsis, 10 g

Caulis Aristolochiae Manshuriensis, 10 g

Bulbus Fritillariae Unibracteatae, 10 g

Radix Glycyrrhizae, 6 g

plain spirits, 200 ml

**Process**   Make decoction with the above ingredients (including plain spirits) in 200 ml of water until 200 ml of decoction retained. Filter the decoction and put the extracts in a bowl for future administration.

**Directions**   Take one half of the decoction warmly, twice daily.

**Indication**   Primary mastitis.

**Recipe** 3

**Ingredients**

Semen Vaccariae, 30 g

Herba Taraxaci, 15 g

Fructus Trichosanthis, 15 g

Radix Angelicae Sinensis, 9 g

plain spirits, 400 ml

**Process**   Make decoction with the above ingredients (in plain spirits) until 200 ml of the decoction retained.

**Directions**   Take one third of the decoction three times daily.

**Indication**   Primary mastitis manifested by aversion to cold and fever.

**Recipe** 4

**Ingredients**

Herba Taraxaci, 10 g

millet wine, 250 ml

**Process**   Wash dandelion herb clean and pound it into mash. Make decoction with the mash in 250 ml of millet wine until it is brought to several times of boils.

**Directions**   Take 20 ml of the decoction with warm soup of Chinese green onion to get mild perspiration, three times daily. Apply the warm dregs on the affected part.

**Indication**   Primary mastitis manifested by distending pain in the breast, difficulty in milk ejection.

## Section 6    Angiitis

Angiitis refers to a patchy inflammation of the walls of small blood vessels. It may result from a variety of conditions, including polyarteritis nodosa, acute nephritis, and serum sickness. Symptoms include skin rashes, arthritis, purpura, and kidney failure.

**Recipe**
**Ingredients**
Radix Salviae Miltiorrhizae, 30 g
plain spirits, 500 ml
**Process**    Wash Dan-Shen root clean and cut into pieces. Soak them in plain spirits and seal the container for 15 days. Shake the container once daily during the soaking time.
**Directions**    Take 20 ml before meals thee times daily.
**Indication**    Thromboangiitis obliterans.

## Section 7    Hernia

Hernia refers to the protrusion of an organ or tissue out of the body cavity in which it normally lies. An inguinal hernia (or rupture) occurs in the lower abdomen; a sac of peritoneum, containing fat or part of the bowel, bulges through a weak part (inguinal canal) of the abdominal wall. It may result from physical straining or coughing. A scrotal hernia is an inguinal hernia so large that it passes into the scrotum; a femoral hernia is similar to an inguinal hernia but protrudes at the point at which the femoral artery passes from the abdomen to the thigh. A diaphragmatic hernia (prescriptions indicated for this condition not discussed here) is the protrusion of an abdominal organ through the diaphragm into the chest cavity; the most common type is the hiatus hernia, in which the stomach passes partly or completely into the chest cavity through the hole (hiatus) for the esophagus (gullet). An umbilical hernia, most common in young children, appears as a bulge at the navel. Hernias may be complicated by becoming impossible to return to their normal site (irreducible); swollen and fixed within their sac (incarcerated); or cut off from their blood supply gangrenous (strangulated). The best treatment for hernias, especially if they are painful, is surgical repair.

**Recipe** 1
**Ingredients**
Fructus foenicuii, 9 g
Semen Persicae, 9 g
millet wine, right amount
**Process**    Soak common fennel fruit and peach kernel in a right amount of millet wine and seal

the container for 15 days.

**Directions** Take the dregs and 10 ml of the tincture for the first time. Then take 5 ml twice daily.

**Indication** Hernia of small intestine.

**Recipe** 2
**Ingredients**
Semen Citri Reticulatae, 20 g
Fructus Foenicuii, 20 g
millet wine, right amount

**Process** Stir-fry common fennel fruit and tangerine seed, grind them into fine powder and mix it equally.

**Directions** Take 5 g of the powder with warm millet wine at bed time, daily.

**Indication** Hernia manifested by painful and swollen testis.

**Recipe** 3
**Ingredients**
Semen Litchi, 9 g
Semen Longan, 9 g
Fructus Foenicuii, 9 g
Rhizoma Cimicifugae, 3 g
plain spirits

**Process** Grind litchi seed, longan seed and common fennel fruit into fine powder. Make decoction with cimicifuga rhizome in a right amount of plain spirits.

**Directions** Take 3 g of the powder with warm decoction of cimicifuga rhizome, twice daily.

**Indication** Hernia of small intestine.

## Section 8  Hemorrhoids

Hemorrhoids refer to enlarged (varicose) veins in the wall of the anus (internal hemorrhoids), usually a consequence of prolonged constipation or, occasionally, diarrhea. They most commonly occur at three main points equidistant around the circumference of the anus. Uncomplicated hemorrhoids are seldom painful; pain is usually caused by a fissure. The main symptom is bleeding. Hemorrhoids can be divided into internal, external and mixed types. According to traditional Chinese medicine, it is often caused by internal dry heat due to improper intake of greasy, spicy, hot food and over indulgence of alcohol, or impairment of collaterals due to forceful bowel excretion in case of constipation. Occupational sitting, long time walk, carrying heavy load and deficiency of organs can cause invasion of exogenous pathogenic wind-damp and retention of heat in the interior, leading to downward flowing of damp-heat accumulated in the anus with stasis to result in hemorrhoids.

**Recipe** 1
**Ingredients**
brown sugar, 100 g

plain spirits, 100 ml

**Process**   Soak brown sugar in boiling plain spirits in a bowl over a slow fire. Take the bowl away from fire until the mixture changes into liquid thoroughly. Let it cool and store it up in a bowl.

**Directions**   Take 20 g of the mixture with warm boiled water, twice daily.

**Indication**   Hemorrhoids.

**Recipe** 2
**Ingredients**
Fructus Luffae, 60 g

spirits, right amount

**Process**   Parch luffa fruit with the nature retained. Then grind them into powder.

**Directions**   Take 6 g with a right amount of spirits, twice daily.

**Indication**   Hematochezia due to hemorrhoids.

**Recipe** 3
**Ingredients**
Misgurnus Anguillicaudatus, 100 g

Radix Astragali, 30 g

rice wine, 20 ml

**Process**   Cut loaches open, remove the internal organs and wash them clean. Make decoction with the above ingredients (including rice wine) in 200 ml of water.

**Directions**   Take the loaches and decoction once daily.

**Indication**   Pain due to hemorrhoids accompanied with prolapse of rectum.

## Section 9   Prolapse of Rectum

Prolapse of rectum is very commonly associated with constipation, hemorrhoids etc.. According to traditional Chinese medicine, this condition is due to deficiency of spleen qi and stomach qi leading to failure of supporting the rectum. Prolapse thus occurs.

**Recipe** 1
**Ingredients**
Cipangopaludina Chinensis, 10

Folium Basjoo, right amount

rice wine, right amount

**Process**   Remove the shells of river snails and soak them in rice wine for 5 hours. Then wrap the snails with basjoo leaves.

**Directions**   Apply the snails on umbilicus, back and coccyx and heat them with moxa sticks for 15 minutes respectively, once daily.

**Indication**   Prolapse of rectum.

**Recipe 2**
**Ingredients**
Fructus Foenicuii, 9 g
Bulbus Allii, 9 g
plain spirits, 5 ml

**Process**   Make decoction with common fennel fruit and Chinese green onion in water until it is brought several times of boils.

**Directions**   Take the decoction with warm plain spirits.

**Indication**   Prolapse of rectum.

**Recipe 3**
**Ingredients**
Retinervus Luffae Fructus, 1
Galla Chinensis, 50 g
rice wine, right amount

**Process**   Grind vegetable sponge of luffa and Chinese galls into fine powder.

**Directions**   Take 5 g of the powder with warm rice wine, twice daily.

**Indication**   Prolapse of rectum.

## Section 10   Bi Syndrome

Bi is Chinese concept, which means obstruction. Conditions characterized by the following chief manifestations, such as aching, numbness and heavy sensation involving the limbs, joints and muscles as well as swollen joints and limited movement due to poor circulation as well as obstruction of qi and blood caused by exogenous pathogenic invasion into the channels and collaterals, are called in general the Bi syndrome. This syndrome is commonly seen in the clinic, also bears the characteristics of progressive pain or pain in repeated attacks. The following conditions: arthralgia and myalgia, numbness of the limbs, lumbocrural pain and podalgia belong to the category of Bi syndrome.

### 1. Arthralgia and Myalgia

**Recipe** 1
**Ingredients**
green plum, 100 g
plain spirits, 500 ml
**Process**　Soak green plums in plain spirits and seal the container for 15 days.
**Directions**　Spread the tincture over the affected part.
**Indicatins**　Arthralgia, pain due to sprain of lumbar region, lumbar muscle strain.

**Recipe** 2
**Ingredients**
Cornu Cervi, 30 g
millet wine, right amount
**Process**　Parch deer horn with its nature retained. Grind the parched horn into fine powder.
**Directions**　Take 3 g of the horn with warm millet wine, twice daily.
**Indicatins**　Arthralgia and myalgia.

**Recipe** 3
**Ingredients**
Caulis Spatholobi, 400 g
plain spirits, 1000 ml
**Process**　Soak suberect spatholobus stem in plain spirits and seal the container for 7 days.
**Directions**　Take 10 ml before meals twice daily.
**Indicatins**　Arthralgia and myalgia.

**Recipe** 4
**Ingredients**
Excrementa Bombycum, 90 g
millet wine, 500 ml
**Process**　Stir-fry silkworm excrement to dry. Fill a gauze bag with the dried excrement. Soak the bag in millet wine and seal the container for 7 days. Take out the bag and filter the tincture for future use.
**Directions**　Take 10 ml twice daily.
**Indicatins**　Arthralgia, myalgia, neuralgia, numbness of the limbs.

2. **Lumbocrural Pain**

**Recipe** 1
**Ingredients**
Folium Spinaciae Oleraceae, 500 g
millet wine, right amount

**Process**  Remove the root of spinach and wash it clean. Pound it into mash and extract its juice.
**Directions**  Take the juice with warm millet wine.
**Indication**  Acute lumbar sprain.

### Recipe 2
**Ingredients**
Radix Aconiti, 30 g
plain spirits,, right amount
**Process**  Grind aconite root into fine powder.
**Directions**  Apply the powder on Yongquan(KI1) of both sides with a right amount of plain spirits.
**Indication**  Acute lumbar sprain.

### Recipe 3
**Ingredients**
Semen Luffae
plain spirits
**Process**  Stir-fry luffa seed with their nature retained. Grind the parched seed into fine powder.
**Directions**  Take 10 g of the powder with warm plain spirits. Apply the powder on the affected part and give moxibustion with moxa sticks for 15 minutes, once daily.
**Indication**  Chronic lumbago.

### Recipe 4
**Ingredients**
Radix Polygoni Multiflori, 180 g
Semen Coicis, 120 g
plain spirits, 1000 ml
**Process**  Cut fleeceflower root into slices. Soak them along with coix seed in plain spirits and seal the container for 14 days. Filter the tincture with gauze and store the extracts up in a clean bottle for future use.
**Directions**  Take 10 to 15 ml twice daily.
**Indicatins**  Lumbago, numbness of the limbs, dizziness due to deficiency of blood.

### Recipe 5
**Ingredients**
Semen Coicis, 45 g
Radix Ledebouriellae, 30 g
Radix Achyranthis Bidentatae, 30 g
Cortex Cinnamomi, 30 g

Radix Angelicae Pubescentis, 30 g

Radix Rehmanniae, 30 g

Semen Sojae Nigrum, 75 g

Radix Angelicae Sinensis, 15 g

Semen Ziziphi Spinosae, 15 g

Rhizoma Chuanxiong, 15 g

Radix Salviae Miltiorrhizae, 15 g

Radix Aconiti Praeparata, 15 g

plain spirits, 1500 ml

**Process**　Stir-fry black soya beans until they become brown. Pound and grind the above ingredients except plain spirits into powder and then fill it a gauze bag. Soak the bag in plain spirits and seal the container for 7 days. Remove the dregs for future use.

**Directions**　Take 10 ml before meals three times daily.

**Indicatins**　Contracture and pain in the lumbar region and knees.

### Recipe 6
**Ingredients**

Radix Achyranthis Bidentatae, 45 g

Rhizoma Dioscoreae Hypoglaucae, 45 g

Radix Aconiti Praeparata, 30 g

Cortex Eucommiae, 30 g

Cortex Cinnamomi, 30 g

Ramulus Loranthi, 30 g

Rhizoma Cibotii, 30 g

Rhizoma et Radix Notoginseng, 30 g

plain spirits, 2500 ml

**Process**　Grind the above ingredients except plain spirits into powder and fill it in a gauze bag. Soak the bag in plain spirits and seal the container for 7 days.

**Directions**　Take 15 ml before meals, twice daily.

**Indicatins**　Lumbocrural pain, contractive sensation of the lower limbs, dyskinesia.

### Recipe 7
**Ingredients**

Rhizoma Cibotii, 30 g

Cortex Eucommiae, 30 g

Rhizoma seu Radix Notopterygii, 30 g

Cortex Cinnamomi, 30 g

Rhizoma Dioscoreae hypoglaucae, 50 g

Radix Aconiti Praeparata, 50 g

Radix Achyranthis Bidentatae, 50 g

Ramulus Loranthi, 40 g

plain spirits, 1500 ml

**Process**  Stir-fry eucommia bark until it becomes yellowish. Pound and grind the above ingredients except plain spirits into powder. Soak the powder in plain spirits and seal the container for 7 days. Remove the dregs and store the extracts up in a clean bottle for future use.

**Directions**  Take 10 ml before meals three times daily.

**Indicatins**  Lumbago, aching pain and contractive sensation of the lower limbs.

## Recipe 8

**Ingredients**

Pseudosciaena Polyactis, 50 g

Cornu Cervi, 50 g

millet wine, 500 ml

**Process**  Stir-fry the first two ingredients in an earthe nware pot until they become brown. Grind them into powder. Soak the powder in millet wine and seal the container for one month. Remove the dregs and store the extracts up in a clean bottle for future use.

**Directions**  Take 20 to 30 ml three times daily.

**Indicatins**  Lumbago and cold sensation in the knees and lumbar region.

## Recipe 9

**Ingredients**

Semen Astragali Complanati, 300 g

plain spirits, 2000 ml

salt solution (3%), 100 ml

**Process**  Soak flatstem milkvetch seed in salt solution for 24 hours. Then Stir-fry them over a slow fire to dry. Grind them into powder. Soak the powder in plain spirits and seal the container for 12 days. Remove the dregs and store the extracts up in a clean bottle for future use.

**Directions**  Take 20 ml twice daily.

**Indicatins**  Insufficiency of liver yin and kidney essence manifested by soreness and pain in the lumbar region and knees, blurring of vision, emission, premature ejaculation, enuresis, frequency of micturition, leukorrhagia.

## Recipe 10

**Ingredients**

Rhizoma Dioscoreae Nipponicae, 100 g

plain spirits, 500 ml

**Process**  Pound Japanese yams into pieces and soak them in plain spirits, seal the container for 7 days. Shaking the container during the soaking time.

**Directions**  Take 30 ml twice daily.

**Indicatins**  Lumbocrural pain, lumbar sprain, osteoarthrosis deformans endemica.

**Recipe 11**
**Ingredients**
Rhizoma Cibotii, 30 g
Radix Salviae Miltiorrhizae, 30 g
Radix Astragali, 30 g
Radix Angelicae Sinensis, 25 g
Radix Ledebouriellae, 15 g
plain spirits, 1000 ml

**Process**   Grind the above ingredients except plain spirits into powder and fill it in a gauze bag. Soak the bag in plain spirits and seal the container for 15 days.

**Directions**   Take 20 ml twice daily.

**Indicatins**   Lumbocrural pain due to deficiency of liver yin and kidney yin, deficiency of qi and blood, or attacking of wind-damp evil.

**Recipe 12**
**Ingredients**
Fructus Psoraleae, 6 g
plain spirits, right amount

**Process**   Grind psoralea fruit into fine powder and store it up in a clean bottle for future use.

**Directions**   Take 6 g of the powder with a right amount of plain spirits, once daily.

**Indicatins**   Lumbago, lassitude and fatigue, insomnia due to deficiency of kidney yin.

**Recipe 13**
**Ingredients**
Semen Cuscutae, 60 g
Cortex Eucommiae, 30 g
Radix Achyranthis, 30 g
plain spirits, 1000 ml

**Process**   Pound the first three ingredients into pieces and soak them in plain spirits, seal the container for 7 days.

**Directions**   Take 30 ml before meals twice daily.

**Indicatins**   Deficiency of liver yin and kidney yin manifested by aching pain in the lumbar region and knees, listlessness.

**Recipe 14**
**Ingredients**
Herba Dendrobii Nobilis, 60 g
Cortex Eucommiae, 60 g
Radix Salviae Miltiorrhizae, 60 g

Radix Rehmanniae, 60 g

Radix Achyranthis Bidentatae, 120 g

plain spirits, 1500 ml

**Process**  Pound the first five ingredients into pieces and soak them in plain spirits, seal the container for 7 days. Remove the dregs and store the extracts up in a clean bottle for future use.

**Directions**  Take 10 ml three times daily.

**Indicatins**  Lumbago due to deficiency of kidney, arthralgia and myalgia, dyskinesia.

**Recipe 15**

**Ingredients**

Radix Achyranthis Bidentatae, 30 g

Semen Coicis, 30 g

Semen Ziziphi Spinosae, 30 g

Radix Paeoniae Rubra, 30 g

Radix Aconiti Praeparata, 30 g

Rhizoma Zingiberis, 30 g

Herba Dendrobii Nobilis, 30 g

Semen Biotae, 30 g

Radix Glycyrrhizae Praeparata, 20 g

plain spirits, 1500 ml

**Process**  Pound and grind the first nine ingredients into fine powder and mix it equally. Soak the powder in plain spirits and seal the container for 7 days.

**Directions**  Take 15 ml twice daily.

**Indications**  Cold pain in the lumbar region and knees, contractive sensation of the lower extremities, numbness of the arms, loose stools, listlessness.

**Recipe 16**

**Ingredients**

Herba Erodii seu Geranii, 50 g

Caulis Erycibes, 50 g

Ramulus Mori, 50 g

Herba Siegesbeckiae, 50 g

plain spirits, 1000 ml

**Process**  Grind the first four ingredients into powder, soak it in plain spirits and seal the container for 14 days. Remove the dregs and store the extracts up in a clean bottle for future use.

**Directions**  Take 10 ml three times daily.

**Indicatins**  Pain in the lumbar region and knees, arthralgia and numbness of the extremities.

**Recipe 17**

**Ingredients**

Cortex Eucommiae, 50 g

plain spirits, 500 ml

**Process**  Cut eucommia bark into pieces, soak them in plain spirits and seal the container for 10 days. Shake the container once daily during soaking time.

**Directions**  Take 10 ml twice daily.

**Indicatins**  Aching pain in the lumbar region, flaccidity of the lower extremities, dizziness due to deficiency of kidney yin.

**Recipe** 18

**Ingredients**

Cortex Eucommiae, 120 g

Folium Photiniae, 30 g

Rhizoma seu Radix Notopterygii, 60 g

Radix Aconiti Praeparata, 10 g

plain spirits, 3000 ml

**Process**  Pound the first four ingredients into pieces, soak them in plain spirits and seal the container for 7 days. Remove the dregs and store the extracts up in a clean bottle for future use.

**Directions**  Take 20 ml twice daily.

**Indicatins**  Lumbocrural pain which is aggravated by coldness, dyskinesia, lassitude and fatigue due to deficiency of kidney and attacking of wind-cold evil.

**Recipe** 19

**Ingredients**

Semen Phaseoli, 50 g

plain spirits, 100 ml

**Process**  Stir-fry red phaseolus beans until they are done. Mix them with plain spirits equally.

**Directions**  Take 25 g of the beans by chewing carefully, twice daily.

**Indication**  Acute lumbar sprain.

**Recipe** 20

**Ingredients**

Cortex Eucommiae, 30 g

Radix Salviae Miltiorrhizae, 30 g

Rhizoma Chuanxiong, 20 g

rice wine, 750 ml

**Process**  Cut the first three ingredients into pieces, soak them in rice wine and seal the container for 5 days. Remove the dregs and store the extracts up in a clean bottle for future use.

**Directions**  Take 10 ml warmly.

**Indication**  Aching pain in the lumbar region and lower extremities.

**Recipe** 21
**Ingredients**
Ramulus Loranthi, 10 g
plain spirits, right amount
**Process**　Stir-fry loranthus mulberry mistletoe to dry and grind into powder.
**Directions**　Take the powder with a right amount of warm plain spirits, once daily.
**Indicatins**　Lumbocrural pain and dyskinesia due to wind-damp evil affecting the channels and collaterals of the lower extremities.

**Recipe** 22
**Ingredients**
Radix Ledebouriellae, 20 g
Rhizoma Chuanxiong, 20 g
Ramulus Loranthi, 20 g
Radix Angelicae Pubescentis, 30 g
Radix Achyranthis Bidentatae, 30 g
Radix Gentianae Macrophyllae, 30 g
Radix Paeoniae Alba, 30 g
Radix Codonopsis Pilosulae, 30 g
Radix Angelicae Sinensis, 50 g
Radix Rehmanniae, 50 g
Cortex Eucommiae, 50 g
Poria, 40 g
Radix Glycyrrhizae, 15 g
Cortex Cinnamomi, 15 g
Herba Asari Heterotropoidedis, 12 g
plain spirits, 1500 ml
**Process**　Pound the above ingredients except plain spirits into pieces, soak them in plain spirits and seal the container for 14 days. Remove the dregs and store the extracts up in a clean bottle for future use.
**Directions**　Take 10 ml three times daily.
**Indicatins**　Lumbocrural pain aggravated in rainy days, numbness of the extremities.

**Recipe** 23
**Ingredients**
Semen Sojae Nigrum, 200 g
Ramulus Loranthi, 200 g
Radix Dipsaci, 100 g
rice wine, 1500 ml
**Process**　Stir-fry black soya beans until they are done; pound dipsacus root and loranthus mul-

berry mistletoe into pieces. Soak them in rice wine and seal the container for 7 days.

**Directions** Take 10 ml twice daily.

**Indicatins** Lumbocrural pain due to deficiency of liver yin and kidney yin resulting in attacking of wind-damp evil, postpartum lumbago.

### Recipe 24
**Ingredients**
Cortex Eucommiae, 15 g
Fructus Psoraleae, 10 g
Rhizoma Atractylodis, 10 g
Cornu Cervi Degelatinatum, 10 g
plain spirits, 500 g

**Process** Pound the first three ingredients into powder. Soak them along with deglued antler powder in plain spirits and seal the container for 7 days.

**Directions** Take 15 ml twice daily.

**Indicatins** Chronic lumbago, arthralgia.

### Recipe 25
**Ingredients**
Folium Photiniae, 15 g
plain spirits, 500 g

**Process** Cut Chinese photinia leaves into pieces, soak them in plain spirits and seal the container for 7 days. Shake the container frequently during soaking. Then remove the dregs and store the extracts up in a clean bottle for future use.

**Directions** Take 15 ml twice daily. One course consisting of 7 days.

**Indicatins** Lumbago, lassitude and fatigue due to deficiency of kidney qi.

### Recipe 26
**Ingredients**
Fructus Corni, 50 g
plain spirits, 500 ml

**Process** Cut dogwood fruit into pieces, soak them in plain spirits and seal the container for 7 days. Shake the container once other day during soaking. Then remove the dregs and store the extracts up in a clean bottle for future use.

**Directions** Take 10 ml once daily.

**Indicatins** Lumbago accompanied by emission, spontaneous perspiration, or menorrhagia in women.

### Recipe 27
**Ingredients**

Semen Juglandis, 60 g

brown sugar, 30 g

millet wine, 30 ml

**Process**   Make decoction with walnut kernels and millet wine in a right amount of water. After the decoction is done, add in brown sugar and stir the mixture equally.

**Directions**   Take the mixture at bed time.

**Indication**   Acute lumbar sprain.

### Recipe 28
**Ingredients**

Herba Allii Tuberosi, 30 g

millet wine, 100 ml

**Process**   Cut Chinese chives into pieces and decoct them in millet wine until it boils.

**Directions**   Take the decoction warmly, once or twice daily.

**Indication**   Acute lumbar sprain with blood stasis.

### Recipe 29
**Ingredients**

Carapax Trionycis, 30 g

millet wine, right amount

**Process**   Stir-fry tortoise shells with their nature retained. Grind them into powder and store up in a bottle for future use.

**Directions**   Take 3 g with warm millet wine, twice daily.

**Indication**   Shooting pain in the lumbar region due to acute sprain.

### Recipe 30
**Ingredients**

Radix Hemerocalis Immaturus, 10 g

Semen Phaseoli, 30 g

millet wine, right amount

**Process**   Make decoction with the root of day lily and red phaseolus beans. After the decoction is done, remove the dregs and add in millet wine.

**Directions**   Take the decoction warmly, once daily.

**Indication**   Swelling pain in the lumbar region due to acute sprain.

## 3. Pain in the Lower Extremities and Podalgia

### Recipe 1
**Ingredients**

Flos Hemerocallis Immaturus, 60 g

crystal sugar, 60 g

millet wine, 100 ml

**Process**   Make decoction with the above ingredients in 500 ml of water until 300 ml of decoction retained.

**Directions**   Take 100 ml of the decoction three times daily.

**Indicatins**   Pain in the lower extremities and podalgia.

### Recipe 2
**Ingredients**

Radix Clematidis, 120 g

millet wine, right amount

**Process**   Pound clematis root into pieces, grind them into powder.

**Directions**   Take 20 g of the powder with warm millet wine, twice daily.

**Indication**   Pain in the lower extremities and podalgia.

### Recipe 3
**Ingredients**

Fructus Evodiae, 30 g

millet wine, right amount

**Process**   Grind dried medicinal evodia fruit into powder, bake it until it is hot enough to take effects.

**Directions**   Apply hot powder on the affected part with a right amount of hot millet wine for 30 minutes. Reheat the powder several times during the treatment. One course consisting of 7 days.

**Indicatins**   Pain in the phalangeal joints, podalgia.

### Recipe 4
**Ingredients**

Folium Artemisiae Argyi, 60 g

Rhizoma Zingiberis, 45 g

Bulbus Allii, 9 g

millet wine, right amount

**Process**   Wash the first three ingredients clean and pound them into mash.

**Directions**   Spread the mash over affected part with hot millet wine for 15 minutes, three times daily.

**Indication**   Pain in the lower extremities.

### Recipe 5
**Ingredients**

Fructus Schisandrae Chinensis, 12 g

Resina Olibani, 12 g
Radix Achyranthis Bidentatae, 20 g
plain spirits, right amount

**Process**　Grind the first three ingredients into fine powder.

**Directions**　Apply the powder on the affected area with a right amount of warm plain spirits, then cover the area with a piece of gauze. Change the powder twice daily.

**Indication**　Pain in the foot due to spurs.

### 4. Arthralgia

**Recipe** 1
**Ingredients**
Folium Persicae, 10 g
plain spirits, 150 ml

**Process**　Pound peach leaves into mash.

**Directions**　Apply the mash on affected part at bed time. 5 minutes later, wash the area with warm plain spirits. Once daily.

**Indication**　Rheumatic arthritis.

**Recipe** 2
**Ingredients**
Zaocys, 1
plain spirits, right amount

**Process**　Soak black-tail snake in plain spirits and seal the container for 2 weeks.

**Directions**　Take 10 to 30 ml twice daily.

**Indication**　Rheumatic arthritis.

**Recipe** 3
**Ingredients**
Rhizoma Zingiberis, 30 g
Bulbus Allii, 30 g
Herba Coriandri, 30 g
Rhizoma Acori Graminei, 15 g
plain spirits, right amount

**Process**　Cut the first four ingredients into pieces, stir-fry them with plain spirits. Fill a gauze bag with the hot pieces.

**Directions**　Apply the hot bag on the diseased region for 15 minutes, three times daily. Reheat the bag during the treatment.

**Indication**　Rheumatic arthritis.

### Recipe 4
**Ingredients**
Folium Pini, 1500 ml
plain spirits, 1250 ml
**Process**  Soak pine leaves in plain spirits and seal the container for 7 days.
**Directions**  Take 10 ml three times daily.
**Indication**  Rheumatic arthritis.

### Recipe 5
**Ingredients**
Radix Rubiae, 15 g
Lignum Pini Nodi, 15 g
plain spirits, 500 ml
**Process**  Soak rubia root and nodular branch of pine in plain spirits, seal the container for 7 days.
**Directions**  Take 10 ml three times daily.
**Indication**  Rheumatoid arthritis.

### Recipe 6
**Ingredients**
Fructus Lycii, 30 g
Cortex Eucommiae, 30 g
Cortex Acanthopanacis Radicis, 30 g
plain spirits, 1500 ml
**Process**  Soak the first ingredients in plain spirits, seal the container for 7 days.
**Directions**  Take 25 ml at bedtime, daily.
**Indication**  Rheumatic arthritis.

### Recipe 7
**Ingredients**
Fructus Psoraleae, 30 g
Semen Juglandis, 60 g
Cortex Eucommiae, 30 g
rice wine, 500 ml
**Process**  Pound the first two ingredients into pieces, soak them along with eucommia bark in rice wine, seal the container for 7 days.
**Directions**  Take 10 ml twice daily.
**Indication**  Rheumatoid arthritis.

**Recipe** 8
**Ingredients**
Radix Clematidis, 500 g

plain spirits, 1500 ml

**Process**  Cut clematis root into pieces, put them along with plain spirits in an earthenware pot. Cover the lid of the pot and steam it in boiling water for half one hour. Remove the dregs and store the extracts for future use.

**Directions**  Take 10 to 20 ml three times daily.

**Indication**  Rheumatic arthritis.

**Recipe** 9
**Ingredients**
Caulis Erycibes, 240 g

Herba Ephedrae, 40 g

Ramulus Cinnamomi, 20 g

Radix Clematidis, 20 g

Radix Angelicae Dahuricae, 20 g

Semen Artemisiae, 20 g

Fructus Foenicuii, 15 g

Radix Stephaniae Tetrandrae, 15 g

Rhizoma seu Radix Notopterygii, 15 g

Radix Angelicae Pubescentis, 15 g

Cortex Acanthopanacis Radicis, 15 g

Radix Angelicae Sinensis, 12.5 g

Rhizoma Chuanxiong, 12.5 g

Fructus Gardeniae, 12.5 g

plain spirits, 2400 ml

**Process**  Put the above ingredients except plain spirits in an earthenware pot. Cover the lid of the pot and steam the ingredients in boiling water until they are done. After it cools, add plain spirits in and seal the pot for 45 days. Shake the pot once other day during soaking.

**Directions**  Take 15 ml twice daily.

**Indications**  Rheumatic arthritis of wind type manifested by wandering arthralgia, numbness of the limbs, dyskinesia, etc..

**Recipe** 10
**Ingredients**
Radix Angelicae Pubescentis, 9 g

Rhizoma Chuanxiong, 9 g

Radix Rehmanniae Praeparata, 9 g

Cortex Eucommiae, 18 g

Radix Angelicae Sinensis, 18 g

Radix Salviae Miltiorrhizae, 20 g

rice wine, 2000 ml

**Process** Pound and grind the above ingredients except rice wine into powder, fill in a gauze bag, soak it in rice wine, seal the container for 5 to 7 days. Remove the bag and dregs and store the extracts up in a clean bottle for future use.

**Directions** Take 20 ml twice daily.

**Indications** Rheumatic arthritis manifested by numbness and cold pain in the waist and lower extremities.

**Recipe 11**

**Ingredients**

Herba Erodii seu Geranii, 50 g

plain spirits, 500 ml

**Process** Pound and grind herb of common heron's bill into powder, soak it in plain spirits, seal the container for 14 days. Shake the container frequently while soaking. Remove the dregs and store the extracts up in a clean bottle for future use.

**Directions** Take 15 ml twice daily.

**Indications** Rheumatic arthritis, traumatic injury.

**Recipe 12**

**Ingredients**

Fructus Chaenomelis, 35 g

Radix Achyranthis, 25 g

plain spirits, 700 ml

**Process** Soak chaenomeles fruit and achyranthes root in plain spirits, seal the container for 15 days. Shake the container frequently while soaking. Remove the dregs and store the extracts up in a clean bottle for future use.

**Directions** Take 10 to 15 ml twice daily.

**Indications** Rheumatic arthritis, ankylosis, dyskinesia.

**Recipe 13**

**Ingredients**

Fructus Chaenomelis, 160 g

Rhizoma Curcumae Longae, 80 g

Rhizoma seu Radix Notopterygii, 80 g

plain spirits, 1100 ml

**Process** Cut the first three ingredients into pieces, soak them in plain spirits, seal the container for 10 days. Shake the container frequently while soaking. Remove the dregs and store the extracts up in a clean bottle for future use.

**Directions**  Take 10 ml three times daily.
**Indication**  Contractive pain in rheumatic arthritis.

**Recipe** 14
**Ingredients**
Caulis Trachelospermi, 45 g
Caulis Piperis Futokadsurae, 45 g
Caulis Spatholobi, 45 g
Ramulus Loranthi, 45 g
Fructus Chaenomelis, 30 g
Cortex Acanthopanacis Radicis, 15 g
plain spirits, 1600 ml
**Process**  Cut the first six ingredients into thin slices, fill them in a gauze, fasten the mouth of it, soak it in plain spirits, seal the container for 21 days. Shake the container frequently while soaking. Remove the bag and dregs and store the extracts up in a clean bottle for future use.
**Directions**  Take 15 ml once daily.
**Indications**  Rheumatic arthritis, arthralgia.

**Recipe** 15
**Ingredients**
Caulis Sinomenii, 15 g
plain spirits, 600 ml
**Process**  Cut orientavine into pieces, soak them in plain spirits, seal the container for 7 days. Shake the container once daily while soaking. Remove the dregs and store the extracts up in a clean bottle for future use.
**Directions**  Take 15 ml twice daily.
**Indications**  Rheumatic arthritis, numbness of the limbs, beriberi marked by palpitation, shortness of breath, edema, oliguria.

**Recipe** 16
**Ingredients**
Rhizoma Homalomenae, 10 g
plain spirits, 600 ml
**Process**  Cut homalomena rhizome into pieces, soak them in plain spirits, seal the container for 7 days. Shake the container once daily while soaking. Remove the dregs and store the extracts up in a clean bottle for future use.
**Directions**  Take 15 ml twice daily.
**Indications**  Rheumatic arthritis, arthralgia, lassitude and fatigue.

**Recipe** 17
**Ingredients**

Herba Aristolochiae Mollissimae, 15 g

plain spirits, 500 g

**Process**  Pound and grind hairy birthwort into powder, soak it in plain spirits, seal the container for 7 days. Shake the container once daily while soaking. Remove the dregs and store the extracts up in a clean bottle for future use.

**Directions**  Take 10 ml before meals, three times daily.

**Indications**  Arthralgia, numbness of the limbs, contracture or contractive sensation of the limbs.

**Recipe 18**

**Ingredients**

Lignum Pini Nodi, 30 g

plain spirits, 500 ml

**Process**  Pound and grind nodular branch of pine into powder, soak it in plain spirits, seal the container for 7 days. Shake the container once daily while soaking. Remove the dregs and store the extracts up in a clean bottle for future use.

**Directions**  Take 15 ml twice daily.

**Indications**  Rheumatic arthritis, arthralgia.

**Recipe 19**

**Ingredients**

Cortex Eucommiae, 15 g

Rhizoma Zingiberis, 15 g

Rhizoma Dioscoreae, 15 g

Radix Aconiti Praeparata, 15 g

Semen Zanthoxyli, 15 g

Cortex Cinnamomi, 15 g

Rhizoma Chuanxiong, 15 g

Rhizoma seu Radix Notopterygii, 15 g

Radix Ledebouriellae, 15 g

Radix Gentianae Macrophyllae, 15 g

Radix Glycyrrhizae, 15 g

Herba Asari Heterotropoidedis, 7.5 g

Cortex Acanthopanacis Radicis, 7.5 g

Herba Dendrobii Nobilis, 7.5 g

Radix Dipsaci, 7.5 g

Cortex Lycii Radicis, 7.5 g

Radix Platycodi, 17 g

plain spirits, 1600 ml

**Process**  Stir-fry bunge pricklyash seed until they are done, pound and grind the first 17 ingredients into powder, put it in an earthenware pot, add in plain spirits, cover the lid, cook it over fire for 4 hours. After it cools, remove the dregs and store the extracts for future use.

**Directions**  Take 10 ml three times daily.

**Indications**  Rheumatic arthritis, arthralgia due to deficiency of kidney yang and attacking of cold-damp evil.

**Recipe** 20
**Ingredients**
Radix Achyranthis Bidentatae, 37.5 g
Radix Gentianae Macrophyllae, 37.5 g
Radix Asparagi, 37.5 g
Radix Angelicae Pubescentis, 45 g
Cortex Cinnamomi, 30 g
Cortex Acanthopanacis Radicis, 30 g
Herba Asari Heterotropoidedis, 15 g
Folium Photiniae, 15 g
Semen Coicis, 15 g
Radix Aconiti Praeparata, 15 g
Radix Morindae Officinalis, 15 g
Cortex Eucommiae, 15 g
plain spirits, 5000 ml

**Process**  Pound and grind the first twelve ingredients into powder, fill it in a gauze bag, soak it in plain spirits, seal the container for 7 to 14 days.

**Directions**  Take 15 ml three times daily.

**Indications**  Rheumatic arthritis, arthralgia aggravated by attacking of cold, numbness of the limbs, dyskinesia.

## 5. Numbness of the Extremities

**Recipe** 1
**Ingredients**
Herba Epimedii, 60 g
plain spirits, 500 ml

**Process**  Fill a gauze bag with epimedium, soak it in plain spirits and seal the container. It can be taken after it has been soaked for three days.

**Directions**  To be taken at bedtime, 10 to 15 ml each time.

**Indication**  Numbness of the extremities.

**Recipe** 2
**Ingredients**

Rhizoma Gastrodiae, 30 g

plain spirits, 500 ml

**Process**　Soak the gastrodia tuber in spirits and seal the container for 7 days.

**Directions**　Take 10 to 20 ml twice daily.

**Indications**　Numbness of the extremities, arthralgia.

### Recipe 3
**Ingredients**

Auricularia, 50 g

Semen Persicae, 15 g

Mel, 50 ml

spirits, 60 ml

**Process**　Have the edible fungus soaked in boiling water and then washed clean. Pound the fungus along with peach kernels into mash. Mix Mel and spirits with the mash equally and then steam the mixture until it is done.

**Directions**　Take it once daily.

**Indication**　Numbness of the extremities due to attacking of wind and damp evil.

### Recipe 4
**Ingredients**

egg shell, 120 g

millet wine, right amount

**Process**　Grind the dried shell into fine powder.

**Directions**　Take 6 g of the powder with warm millet wine, twice daily.

**Indications**　Pain and numbness of the extremities.

### Recipe 5
**Ingredients**

Radix Asparagi, 60 g

white spirits, 500 ml

**Process**　Have lucid asparagus clean. Fill a gauze bag with lucid sparagus and then soak it in spirits and seal the container for 30 days.

**Directions**　Take 20 to 30 ml once daily.

**Indications**　Pain and numbness of the extremities.

### Recipe 6
**Ingredients**

Radix Rehmanniae, 60 g

spirits, 500 ml

**Process**　Have dried rehmannia root clean. Fill a gauze bag with rehmanniae root and then soak it in spirits and seal the container for 7 days.

**Directions**   Take 5 ml before sleep once daily.

**Indications**   Pain and numbness of the extremities due to deficiency of yin and blood resulting in malnutrition of the muscles.

**Recipe 7**
**Ingredients**
Semen Sojae Nigrum, 250 g

millet wine, 500 ml

**Process**   Stir-fry the black soya beans until they are done. Soak them in millet wine and seal the container for 7 days. Then remove the dregs for later use.

**Directions**   Take 10 ml after meals twice daily.

**Indications**   Pain and numbness of the extremities due to deficiency of blood and attacking of wind evil.

## Section 11   Sciatica

Sciatica is a kind of radiating and continuous pain in the course of sciatic nerve distribution, i. e. pain in the hip region, the posterolateral aspect of the thigh and leg, and lateral aspect of the foot. According to its etiology, sciatica can be divided into the primary and secondary types. Sciatic neuritis, the primary type, is caused mainly by pathological stimulation, pressing or injuring of the adjacent nerves affecting the sciatic nerve. This is also clinically known as symptomatic sciatica. The secondary sciatica is more common than the primary. Primary sciatica is characterized by a sudden onset of continuous sharp pain that aggravates in paroxysmal attacks. The paroxysmal pain, burning and sharp in nature, worsens with cold, but alleviates with warmth. There may appear some points of tenderness along the sciatic nerve. Stretching and raising of leg tests are positive. An increase of ankle flexing is seen in the early stage, but decreases in the later stage without apparent muscular atrophy.

Secondary sciatica is markedly by a slow onset of pain which may sometimes involve primary lesions. It is mainly a kind of radiating pain due to lumbar disc degeneration. The pain is often worse with cough, sneezing or halting of the breath. Disc and spinal tenderness are involved. Fewer points of tenderness are found along the course of the sciatic nerve. Stretching and raising of legs tests also appear positive. Chin-chest and Queckenstedt's tests appear positive but ankle flexing is mostly decreasing, or disappearing in the severe case. There will be muscular atrophy in the severe case.

**Recipe 1**
**Ingredients**
Concha Haliotidis, 9 g

Periostracum Serpentis, 9 g

Herba Menthae, 9 g

millet wine, right amount

**Process**  Grind the first two ingredients into powder. Make decoction with peppermint in millet wine.

**Directions**  Take the powder with the decoction, once daily.

**Indication**  Sciatica.

### Recipe 2

**Ingredients**

Corium Erinacei, 100 g

millet wine, right amount

**Process**  Bake hedgehog skin until it becomes brown. Grind it into powder and store up in a bottle for future use.

**Directions**  Take 10 of the powder twice daily. One course consisting of 5 days.

**Indication**  Sciatica.

### Recipe 3

**Ingredients**

Ramulus Cinnamomi, 15 g

Radix Achyranthis Bidentatae, 15 g

Radix Clematidis, 15 g

Radix Dipsaci, 15 g

Semen Persicae, 15 g

Caulis Piperis Futokadsurae, 15 g

Resina Olibani, 15 g

Myrrha, 15 g

Scorpio, 5 g

plain spirits, 2000 ml

**Process**  Soak the above ingredients except plain spirits into powder, soak them in plain spirits and seal the container for one week.

**Directions**  Take the tincture and dregs with 10 days.

**Indication**  Sciatica.

### Recipe 4

**Ingredients**

Herba Siegesbeckiae, 1000 g

Ramulus Mori, 1500 g

plain spirits, 250 ml

**Process**  Make decoction with mulberry twigs and siegesbeckia herbs in water until 250 ml of decoction retained. After it cools, add 250 ml of plain spirits in the decoction and store the mixture up in a bottle for later use.

**Directions**  Take 20 to 25 ml three times daily. One course consisting of 7 days.

**Indication**  Sciatica.

**Recipe** 5
**Ingredients**
Flos Impatientis, 200 g
millet wine, 600 ml

**Process**  Bake garden balsam flower to dry, then grind them into powder. Soak it in millet wine for 7 days. Remove the dregs and store the extracts up in a bottle for future use.

**Directions**  Take 15 ml twice daily.

**Indications**  Lumbago, chronic rheumatic arthritis.

**Recipe** 6
**Ingredients**
Cortex Acanthopanacis Radicis, 100 g
plain spirits, 1000 ml

**Process**  Cut acanthopanax bark into pieces, soak them in plain spirits and seal the container for 25 to 30 days. Remove the dregs and store the extracts up in a bottle for future use.

**Directions**  Take 10 ml twice daily.

**Indication**  Aching pain in the waist and lower limbs due to attacking of wind-cold and damp evil.

## Section 12    Fracture

The following prescriptions are effective for improving the symptoms especially for alleviating the pains resulted from fracture.

**Recipe** 1
**Ingredients**
Herba Allii Tuberosi, 60 g
Bulbus Allii, 30 g
Lumbricus, 20 g
plain spirits, right amount

**Process**  Pound Chinese chives, Chinese green onion and earthworms into mash.

**Directions**  Apply the mash on the affected part with a right amount of plain spirits.

**Indication**  Fracture.

**Recipe** 2
**Ingredients**
Crab, 1
millet wine, right amount
**Process**　Bake the crab to dry and grind it into fine powder.
**Directions**　Take 9 to 12 g of the powder with warm millet wine orally, twice daily.
**Indication**　Fracture.

**Recipe** 3
**Ingredients**
Radix Notoginseng, 50 g
Eupolyphaga seu Steleophaga, 50 g
Pericarpium Citri Reticulatae, 30 g
millet wine, right amount
**Process**　Bake the first three ingredients to dry and grind them into fine powder.
**Directions**　Take 10 g of the powder with a right amount of millet wine, three times daily.
**Indication**　Fracture.

**Recipe** 4
**Ingredients**
Rhizoma Drynariae, 60 g
plain spirits, 500 ml
**Process**　Soak drynaria rhizome in plain spirits and seal the container for 7 days. Remove the dregs and store the extracts up in a bottle for future use.
**Directions**　Take 10 ml twice daily.
**Indication**　Fracture.

**Recipe** 5
**Ingredients**
Semen Phaseoli Radiati, 30 g
Eupolyphaga seu Steleophaga, 20 g
millet wine, right amount
**Process**　Grind mung beans into fine powder and stir-fry it until it becomes purplish. Bake ground beetles until they become yellowish and then grind them into powder.
**Directions**　Apply the powder of mung beans on the affected part with a right amount of millet wine, then bind up the area with gauze. In the mean time, take the powder of ground beetles with warm millet wine orally, once daily.
**Indication**　Fracture.

# Section 13  Scapulohumeral Periarthritis

Scapulohumeral periarthritis, also known as frozen shoulder, is a condition that bothers most of its victims at the age around fifty. It is characterized by a heavy aching on one or two shoulders and limited movement. Frozen shoulder is mostly caused by weakness of the nutrient and defensive systems, asthenia of muscles and joints as well as wind-cold invasion. However, twisting and contusion due to careless exertion or stagnation of qi and blood due to habitual onesided sleep pressing the channels and collaterals may also cause frozen shoulder.

**Recipe** 1
**Ingredients**
Ramulus Pini, 2500 g
plain spirits, 5000 ml
**Process**　　Soak pine twigs in plain spirits and seal the container for 7 days. Then remove the dregs and store the extracts up in a bottle for future use.
**Directions**　　Take 30 ml after meals, twice daily.
**Indication**　　·Scapulohumeral periarthritis.

**Recipe** 2
**Ingredients**
pork, 250 g
Agaricus Campestris, 250 g
Pericarpium Zanthoxyli, 5 g
millet wine, 30 ml
plain spirits, 30 ml
**Process**　　Make decoction with bunge pricklyash peel in 30 ml of water. Cut pork into slices and mix them with mushrooms in an earthenware pot. Add millet wine and the decoction of bunge pricklyash peel in the pot, cover the lid, steam them in boiling water until they are done.
**Directions**　　Take one half of the pork and mushrooms with plain spirits, twice daily.
**Indication**　　Scapulohumeral periarthritis.

**Recipe** 3
**Ingredients**
Radix Clematidis, 15 g
Rhizoma Atractylodis, 15 g
Radix Ledebouriellae, 15 g
Excrementa Bombycum, 30 g
millet wine, 120 ml

**Process**  Stir-fry the first three ingredients to dry, then add in 120 ml of millet wine, go on stir-frying for a few minutes. Then fill them in a gauze bag.

**Directions**  Apply the bag on affected part for 30 minutes, while it is hot. The bag should be reheated every 10 minutes.

**Indication**  Scapulohumeral periarthritis.

### Recipe 4
**Ingredients**

Rhizoma Zingiberis, 1000 g

Bulbus Allii, 500 g

millet wine, 250 ml

**Process**  Pound old ginger and Chinese green onion into mash. Stir-fry the mash along with millet wine until the mash is hot enough to take effects.

**Directions**  Apply the mash on affected part and change the mash twice daily. One course consisting of 7 days.

**Indications**  Scapulohumeral periarthritis, scapulalgia.

### Recipe 5
**Ingredients**

Folium Eriobotryae, 10 g

Folium Artemisiae Argyi, 10 g

Rhizoma Zingiberis, 10 g

millet wine, 10 ml

**Process**  Wash the first three ingredients clean, pound them into mash. Stir-fry the mash along with millet wine until it is hot enough to take effects.

**Directions**  Apply the mash on affected part and change it twice daily. One course consisting of 7 days.

**Indication**  Intractable scapulohumeral periarthritis.

## Section 14  Traumatic Injury

Trauma is very commonly seen in productive labor and daily life, mainly including incised wound, punctured wound, stabbed wound, impacted wound and so on. As far as the locations of injury are concerned, some are in the joints of the limbs, some in the waist, and some in certain other parts of the body.

The subsequent prescription can be applied for cases with various kinds of symptoms resulting from traumatic injury.

**Recipe** 1
**Ingredients**
Radix Angelicae Sinensis, 45 g
Fructus Lycii, 45 g.
Radix Notoginseng, 30 g
Cortex Eucommiae, 30 g
Radix Rehmanniae Praeparata, 30 g
Os Tigris, 30 g
Fructus Chaenomelis, 30 g
Cortex Acanthopanacis Radicis, 30 g
Radix Dipsaci, 23 g
Lignum Aquilariae Resinatum, 7.5 g
Radix Astragali, 22 g
Radix Ginseng Alba, 15 g
Radix Polygoni Multiflori, 15 g
Rhizoma seu Radix Notopterygii, 15 g
Radix Angelicae Pubescentis, 15 g
Stigma Croci, 4.5 g
crystal sugar, 250 g
plain spirits, 2500 ml

**Process** Pound the above ingredients except crystal sugar and plain spirits into powder. Soak the powder in plain spirits and seal the container, put it in a cool, dry place for 15 days. Mix the tincture with crystal sugar equally.

**Directions** Take 30 ml twice daily.

**Indications** Weakness of the muscles after reduction of fracture dislocation.

**Recipe** 2
**Ingredients**
Radix Paeoniae Rubra, 13 g
Radix Angelicae Sinensis, 10 g
Radix Rehmanniae, 8 g
Rhizoma Zedoariae, 8 g
Herba Serissae, 8 g
Rhizoma Sparganii, 8 g
Herba Lycopi, 8 g
Rhizoma Alismatis, 8 g
Rhizoma Chuanxiong, 8 g
Semen Persicae, 8 g

Flos Carthami, 6 g

Lignum Sappan, 6 g

Eupolyphaga seu Steleophaga, 4 g

Radix Notoginseng, 1 g

plain spirits, 1000 ml

**Process**   Pound the above ingredients into powder and soak them in plain spirits and seal the container, put it in a cool, dry place for 45 days. Shake the container once daily during soaking. Filter the tincture and store it up for future administration.

**Directions**   Take 10 ml twice daily.

**Indications**   Traumatic injuries, swelling pain due to blood stasis, sprain of joints, arthralgia, shooting pain in the lumbar region.

**Recipe 3**

**Ingredients**

Semen Persicae, 15 g

Flos Carthami, 15 g

Radix Gentianae Macrophyllae, 15 g

Radix Dipsaci, 15 g

Radix Aucklandiae, 15 g

Fructus Amomi, 15 g

Cortex Moutan Radicis, 15 g

Radix Clematidis, 15 g

Radix Angelicae Sinensis, 45 g

Cortex Acanthopanacis, 45 g

Radix Achyranthis Bidentatae, 45 g

Rhizoma Drynariae, 30 g

Semen Juglandis, 30 g

Cortex Eucommiae, 30 g

Radix Salviae Miltiorrhizae, 30 g

plain spirits, 5000 ml

**Process**   Pound the above ingredients into powder and soak it in 2500 ml of plain spirits in a container. Steam the container in boiling water for 4 hour. Then add the other 2500 ml in and seal the container, put it in a cool, dry place for 3 days. Shake the container once daily during soaking. Filter the tincture and store it up for future administration.

**Directions**   Take 15 ml twice daily.

**Indications**   Myalgia and dyskinesia due to traumatic injuries or hyperkinesia.

**Recipe 4**

**Ingredients**

Flos Caryophylli, 30 g

Radix Angelicae Sinensis, 90 g

Rhizoma Chuanxiong, 90 g

Flos Carthami, 90 g

Radix Notoginseng, 15 g

Flos Impatientis, 45 g

Lignum Sappan, 45 g

Zaocys, 1

plain spirits, 1800 ml

**Process**  Cut the above ingredients except plain spirits into pieces and soak them in plain spirits and seal the container, put it in a cool, dry place for 60 days. Shake the container once daily during soaking. Filter the tincture and store it up for future administration.

**Directions**  Take 15 ml twice daily.

**Indications**  Pain and swelling due to blood stasis resulting from traumatic injury.

**Recipe** 5

**Ingredients**

Flos Impatientis, 10 g

Radix et Rhizoma Rhei, 10 g

Radix Angelicae Sinensis, 10 g

Radix Paeoniae Rubra, 10 g

Gryllotalpa, 10 g

Flos Carthami, 10 g

Eupolyphaga seu Steleophaga, 30 g

Cortex Moutan Radicis, 6 g

Radix Rehmanniae, 15 g

Pyritum, 3 g

spirits, 500 ml

**Process**  Pound ground beetles into mash and grind pyrite into powder. Pound the other ingredients except spirits into pieces and soak them along with the mash in spirits in an earthenware pot. Decoct the ingredients until one half of the decoction left.

**Directions**  Take the powder of pyrite with 1/6 of the decoction once daily. Six days consisted of one course.

**Indications**  Traumatic injury, fracture.

**Recipe** 6

**Ingredients**

Succus Rehmanniae, 250 ml

Cortex Moutan Radicis, 30 g

Cortex Cinnamomi, 30 g

Semen Persicae, 30 g

plain spirits, 500 ml

**Process**　Stir-fry peach kernels until they are done. Pound and grind the ingredients except plain spirits into fine powder. Decoct the powder in rehmannia juice and plain spirits until it is brought to several times of boils. Filter the decoction and store the extracts up in a clean bottle for future use.

**Directions**　Take 10 ml three times daily.

**Indications**　Pain in the abdomen due to blood stasis resulting from trauma.

### Recipe 7
**Ingredients**
Radix Angelicae Sinensis, 6 g
Rhizoma Chuanxiong, 3 g
Flos Carthami, 1.8 g
Radix Rubiae, 1.5 g
Radix Clematidis, 1.5 g
plain spirits, right amount

**Process**　Decoct the above ingredients in a right amount of spirits.

**Directions**　Take the decoction once daily.

**Indications**　Swelling, pain, and dyskinesia due to traumata including subcutaneous tissues, muscles, tendons, fasciae, joint capsules, ligaments, vessels, and peripheral nerves, etc..

### Recipe 8
**Ingredients**
Semen Persicae, 30 g
Succus Rehmanniae, 500 g
plain spirits, 500 g

**Process**　Decoct rehmannia juice in plain spirits until it boils. Pound peach kernel into mash and put it in the decoction and continue decocting the decoction until it is brought to several times of boils. Remove the dregs from the decoction.

**Directions**　Take 10 ml three times daily.

**Indications**　traumata of the muscles.

### Recipe 9
**Ingredients**
Radix Notoginseng, 15 g
Cortex Erythrinae, 15 g
Semen Coicis, 15 g
Rehmanniae, 15 g
Radix Achyranthis, 15 g
Rhizoma Chuanxiong, 15 g
Rhizoma seu Radix Notopterygii, 15 g

Cortex Lycii Radicis, 15 g

Cortex Acanthopanacis Radicis, 15 g

plain spirits, 2500 ml

**Process**  Grind the above ingredients except plain spirits into powder and soak it in plain spirits and seal the container, put it in a cool, dry place for 7 days. Shake the container once daily during soaking. Filter the tincture and store it up for future administration.

**Directions**  Take 15 ml of the tincture twice daily.

**Indications**  Swelling pain due to blood stasis resulting from traumatic injuries.

**Recipe 10**

**Ingredients**

Radix Notoginseng, 15 g

Flos Carthami, 15 g

Radix Rehmanniae, 15 g

Rhizoma Chuanxiong, 15 g

Radix Angelicae Sinensis, 15 g

Radix Linderae, 15 g

Herba Centellae, 15 g

Resina Olibani, 15 g

Cortex Acanthopanacis Radicis, 15 g

Radix Ledebouriellae, 15 g

Radix Cyathulae, 15 g

Rhizoma Zingiberis, 15 g

Cortex Moutan Radicis, 15 g

Cortex Cinnamomi, 15 g

Rhizoma Corydalis, 15 g

Rhizoma Curcumae Longae, 15 g

Cortex Erythrinae, 15 g

plain spirits, 2500 ml

**Process**  Pound the above ingredients except plain spirits into powder. Fill a gauze bag with the powder and soak it in plain spirits in a pot. Cover the basin of the pot and steam it in boiling water for 1.5 hours. Take the bag out, let it cool. Then soak the bag again in plain spirits in the same pot, seal it and put it in a cool, dry place for several days. Shake the container once daily during soaking. Filter the tincture and store it up for future administration.

**Directions**  Take 15 to 20 ml twice daily.

**Indications**  Arthralgia and myalgia and dyskinesia due to stagnation of qi and blood stasis resulting from traumatic injuries.

**Recipe 11**

**Ingredients**

Radix Notoginseng, 45 g

plain spirits, 500 g

**Process**  Cut notoginseng into pieces and put them in an earthenware pot. Add plain spirits in the pot and cover the basin of the pot, make decoction over a slow fire until it boils. Move the pot away from fire and let it cool. Filter the decoction and store the extract in a clean bottle. Seal the bottle for 7 days.

**Directions**  Take 15 ml twice daily.

**Indications**  Traumatic injury, hematemesis due to hyperkinesia, lumbago, general weakness.

## Recipe 12

**Ingredients**

Herba Serissae, 60 g

Rhizoma Drynariae, 60 g

Rhizoma Corydalis, 60 g

plain spirits, 1000 ml

**Process**  Cut serissa, drynaria rhizome and corydalis tuber into pieces. Soak them in plain spirits and seal the container, put it in a cool, dry place for 10 days. Shake the container once daily during soaking. Filter the tincture and store it up for future administration.

**Directions**  Take 10 ml twice daily.

**Indications**  Swelling pain due to blood stasis resulting from traumatic injuries.

## Recipe 13

**Ingredients**

Lignum Sappan, 70 g

plain spirits, 500 ml

**Process**  Pound and grind sappan wood into powder. Put it in an earthenware pot. Add 500 ml of water and 500 ml of plain spirits in the pot and cover the basin, decoct the powder until 500 ml of the decoction retained.

**Directions**  Take 10 ml of the decoction twice daily.

**Indications**  Traumatic injury and swelling pain.

## Recipe 14

**Ingredients**

Flos Impatientis, 90 g

Radix Angelicae Sinensis, 60 g

plain spirits, 1000 ml

**Process**  Soak garden balsam flower and Chinese angelica in plain spirits and seal the container, put it in a cool, dry place for 7 days. Shake the container once daily during soaking. Filter the tincture and store it up for future administration.

**Directions**  Take 30 ml once daily.

**Indications**     Traumata of the muscles, tendons, ligaments and bones.

**Recipe** 15
**Ingredients**
Rhizoma seu Radix Notopterygii, 3 g
Radix Ledebouriellae, 3 g
Cortex Cinnamomi, 3 g
Lignum Sappan, 5 g
Fructus Forsythiae, 6 g
Radix Angelicae Sinensis, 6 g
Radix Bupleuri, 6 g
Hirudo, 9 g
Moschus, 1 g
plain spirits, 1000 ml
**Process**     Grind leeches and musk into mash. Make decoction with the other ingredients except plain spirits in 200 ml of water until 100 ml retained. Filter the decoction and put the extracts and the mash into plain spirits and mix them equally.
**Directions**     Take 15 ml of the mixture before meals, twice daily.
**Indications**     Pain due to blood stasis resulting from traumata.

**Recipe** 16
**Ingredients**
Cipangopaludina Chinensis, 1
Radix Notoginseng, 3 g
millet wine, 10 ml
**Process**     Bake river snail and then grind it into powder. Mix it with powder of notoginseng equally.
**Directions**     Take the powder with warm millet wine.
**Indications**     Traumata.

**Recipe** 17
**Ingredients**
Rhizoma Drynariae, 60 g
plain spirits, 500 ml
**Process**     Soak drynaria rhizome in plain spirits and seal the container, put it in a cool, dry place for 7 days. Filter the tincture and store the extract in a clean bottle for later use.
**Directions**     Take 10 ml twice daily.
**Indications**     Traumata.

### Recipe 18
**Ingredients**
Rhizoma Chuanxiong, 30 g

plain spirits, 500 ml

**Process** Soak Szechuan lovage rhizome in plain spirits and seal the container, put it in a cool, dry place for 7 days. Filter the tincture and store the extracts in a clean bottle for later use.

**Directions** Take 10 ml once daily.

**Indications** Traumata.

### Recipe 19
**Ingredients**
Radix Rosae Rugosae, 25 g

millet wine, right amount

**Process** Make decoction with rose root in a right amount of millet wine.

**Directions** Take one half of the decoction twice daily.

**Indications** Traumata.

### Recipe 20
**Ingredients**
Semen Melo, 9 g

millet wine, 5 ml

**Process** Bake muskmelon seed and grind them into powder.

**Directions** Take the powder warm millet wine, twice daily.

**Indications** sprain of the joints of the extremities.

### Recipe 21
**Ingredients**
Herba Serissae, 30 g

Rhizoma Corydalis, 30 g

Rhizoma Drynariae, 30 g

urine of a boy under 12, 100 ml

plain spirits, 100 ml

**Process** Cut drynaria rhizome, serissa and corydalis tuber into pieces. Make decoction with the pieces in 1000 ml of water until 700 ml retained. Filter the decoction and mix the extracts with urine and spirits equally.

**Directions** Take 20 ml of the mixture with a right amount of warm plain spirits.

**Indications** Traumata with blood stasis in the abdomen.

### Recipe 22
**Ingredients**

Retinervus Luffae Fructus, 30 g

Semen Canavaliae, 30 g

millet wine, 10 ml

**Process**　Parch vegetable sponge of luffa and sword beans with their nature retained. Then grind them into fine powder.

**Directions**　Take 15 g of the powder with warm millet wine, twice daily.

**Indications**　Traumata.

Recipe 23

**Ingredients**

Semen Raphani, 60 g

plain spirits, right amount

**Process**　Pound radish seed into mash, mix it with a right amount of warm plain spirits to make cakes the size of a coin.

**Directions**　Apply the warm medicated cakes on the diseased region.

**Indications**　Swelling pain due to blood stasis resulting from traumata.

Recipe 24

**Ingredients**

Bulbus Allii, 10 g

plain spirits, right amount

**Process**　Pound Chinese green onion into mash.

**Directions**　Apply the mash on the diseased region with warm plain spirits.

**Indications**　Traumata, rheumatalgia.

Recipe 25

**Ingredients**

Fructus Gardeniae, 5 g

plain spirits, right amount

**Process**　Grind cape jasmine fruit into fine powder.

**Directions**　Spread some of the powder over the affected part with a right amount of warm spirits.

**Indications**　Traumata with no external hemorrhage.

Recipe 26

**Ingredients**

Radix Paeoniae Alba, 30 g

plain spirits, 6 g

**Process**　Bake white peony root until it becomes brown. Grind the root into fine powder.

**Directions**　Take 15 g of the powder with water. Apply the other 15 g of powder on the affected part.

**Indications**   Hemorrhage due to traumata.

**Recipe** 27
**Ingredients**
Cornu Bubali, 10 g
plain spirits, right amount

**Process**   Parch buffalo horn with its nature retained. Grind the parched horn into fine powder.

**Directions**   Apply the powder on the affected part with a right amount of plain spirits, once daily.

**Indications**   Hematoma of the muscles due to traumata.

# Chapter Three
# Gynecologic and Obstetric Diseases

## Section 1  Irregular Menstruation

Irregular menstruation refers to abnormal menstrual flow concerning the cycle, duration, color, quantity and quality. They are mainly related to the climatic and environmental changes or emotional disturbances.

1. Preceded menstrual flow: The flow in the case comes earlier than the expected cycle due to mainly the failure of spleen to govern the blood, disharmony between the Chong and Ren Channels, and qi deficiency, or pathogenic heat in blood causing disturbance in the sea of blood so that the flow appears in advance.

2. Delayed menstrual flow: This condition may ascribe to either deficiency or excess factors. The former is caused by deficiency of nutrient blood or that of yang qi; the latter by obstruction of the Chong and Ren Channels due to stagnation of qi and blood, or blood stasis formed cold retention, and impaired circulation of qi and blood between the Chong and Ren Channels, leading to delayed menstrual flow.

3. Disorderly menstrual flow: This condition is mostly caused by impaired circulation of qi and blood due to stagnation of liver qi, deficiency of kidney qi. Common factors such as emotional depression, excessive anger, over consumption of kidney qi due to excessive sex or grand multiparity may lead to disharmony between the Chong and Ren Channels, resulting in a disorderly menstrual flow.

**Recipe 1**
**Ingredients**
Radix Paeoniae Alba, 100 g
Radix Astragali, 100 g
Radix Rehmanniae, 100 g
Folium Artemisiae Argyi, 30 g
plain spirits, 1000 ml

**Process**  Stir-fry argyi leaves until they are done. Pound and grind the first four ingredients into powder, fill it in a gauze bag, soak it in plain spirits and seal the container for 24 hours.

**Directions**  Take 20 ml of the tincture before meals, two times daily.

**Indications**  Menorrhagia, leukorrhagia, leukorrhea with bloody discharge.

**Recipe 2**
**Ingredients**
Radix Sanguisorbae, 62 g

rice wine, right amount

**Process**  Grind sanguisorba root into fine powder and make decoction with it in 100 ml of rice wine until 50 ml of decoction is retained.

**Directions**  Take 15 ml of the decoction twice daily.

**Indications**  Menorrhagia, distending pain in the abdomen and waist, irritability.

### Recipe 3
**Ingredients**

Fructus Foenicuii, 15 g

Pericarpium Citri Reticulatae Viride, 15 g

millet wine, 250 ml

**Process**  Wash common fennel fruit and green tangerine orange peel clean, soak them in millet wine, seal the container for 3 days.

**Directions**  Take 15 ml twice daily.

**Indications**  Irregular menstrual cycle, distending pain in the lower abdomen and breast radiating to the hypochondria, chest distress.

### Recipe 4
**Ingredients**

Flos Carthami, 15 g

Fructus Crataegi, 30 g

plain spirits, 250 ml

**Process**  Soak safflower and hawthorn fruit in spirits and seal the container for one week.

**Directions**  Take 15 ml once daily.

**Indications**  Scanty menses of purplish color with clots in it, dysmenorrhea due to blood stasis.

### Recipe 5
**Ingredients**

Herba Leonuri, 200 g

Radix Angelicae Sinensis, 100 g

plain spirits, 1000 ml

**Process**  Pound and grind the first two ingredients into powder, soak it in plain spirits and seal the container for 7 days.

**Directions**  Take 20 ml once daily.

**Indication**  Amenorrhea due to deficiency of blood.

### Recipe 6
**Ingredients**

Excrementa Bombycum, 120 g

millet wine, 600 ml

**Process**   Stir-fry silkworm excrement until it becomes yellowish, soak it in millet wine in an earthenware pot, cover the lid, cook the lid in water over a slow fire for one hour.

**Directions**   Take 20 ml once daily.

**Indications**   Amenorrhea, arthralgia, numbness of the limbs.

## Recipe 7
**Ingredients**
Fructus Amomi, 30 g
Fructus Citri, 30 g
Fructus Crataegi, 30 g
millet wine, 500 ml

**Process**   Wash the first three ingredients clean, soak them in millet wine and seal the container for 3 to 6 days.

**Directions**   Take 15 ml once daily.

**Indications**   Delayed menstrual cycles, scanty menses with clots, distention in the abdomen and breast radiating to the hypochondria, and mental depression during menstrual periods.

## Recipe 8
**Ingredients**
Radix Achyranthis Bidentatae, 60 g
Radix Codonopsis Pilosulae, 30 g
Radix Angelicae Sinensis, 30 g
Rhizoma Cyperi, 30 g
Flos Carthami, 18 g
Cortex Cinnamomi, 18 g
plain spirits, 1000 ml

**Process**   Cut the first six ingredients into small cubes, soak them in plain spirits, seal the container for 7 days.

**Directions**   Take 10 ml twice daily.

**Indications**   Amenorrhea accompanied with distending pain or cold pain in the lower abdomen, aching pain in the lumbar region, dusty complexion.

## Recipe 9
**Ingredients**
Radix et Rhizoma Rhei, 60 g
plain spirits, right amount

**Process**   Grind rhubarb into powder and store it up for future use.

**Directions**   Take 3 g with a right amount of plain spirits, once daily.

**Indications**   Delayed menstrual cycles due to blood stasis obstructing the collaterals, dysmenorrhea, scanty menses with clots.

**Recipe 10**
**Ingredients**
Radix Salviae Miltiorrhizae, 60 g

plain spirits, 1000 ml

**Process**  Wash Dan-Shen root clean, cut into thin slices, dry them in the sun, then fill them in a gauze bag, fasten the mouth, soak it in plain spirits, seal the container for 15 days.

**Directions**  Take 15 ml twice daily.

**Indications**  Irregular menstruation, thromboangiitis obliterans, angina pectoris.

**Recipe 11**
**Ingredients**
Caulis Spatholobi, 60 g

crystal sugar, 40 g

plain spirits, 500 ml

**Process**  Cut suberect spatholobus stem into thin slices, make decoction with them in plain spirits over a slow fire until it boils. After it cools, seal the container for 5 days. Filter the decoction with a piece of gauze and mix the extracts with dissolved crystal sugar equally. Store the mixture up in a clean bottle for future use.

**Directions**  Take 15 ml once daily.

**Indication**  Delayed menstrual cycles.

**Recipe 12**
**Ingredients**
Radix Angelicae Sinensis, 30 g

Cortex Cinnamomi, 6 g

rice wine, 500 ml

**Process**  Soak the first two ingredients in rice wine and seal the container for six to seven days.

**Directions**  Take 15 ml once daily.

**Indication**  Delayed menstrual cycles.

**Recipe 13**
**Ingredients**
Radix Salviae Miltiorrhizae, 30 g

Rhizoma Chuanxiong, 12 g

Radix Polygoni Multiflori, 12 g

Radix Glycyrrhizae, 12 g

Poria cum Ligno Hospite, 12 g

Fructus Lycii, 9 g

Fructus Schisandrae Chinensis, 9 g

Fructus Amomi Rotundus, 9 g
Cornu Cervi Pantotrichum, 6 g
Rhizoma Atractylodis Macrocephalae, 15 g
Semen Nelumbinis, 15 g
Radix Polygalae, 15 g
Radix Rehmanniae, 15 g
Radix Angelicae Sinensis, 15 g
Rhizoma Anemones Altaicae, 15 g
white sugar, 250 g
plain spirits, 2500 ml

**Process** Fill the above ingredients except plain spirits in a gauze bag, fasten its mouth and soak it in plain spirits in a pot, dissolve white sugar in it, cover the lid and steam the pot in boiling water for 3 hours. After it cools, seal the container and put it in a cool, dark place for 5 days. Then remove the bag and store the extracts up for future use.

**Directions** Take 15 ml twice daily.

**Indications** Metrorrhagia, metrostaxis, irregular menstrual cycles, amenorrhea due to stagnation of qi and blood stasis, leukorrhagia, leukorrhea with bloody discharge, soreness of the waist and lower extremities, consumption.

### Recipe 14
**Ingredients**
Flos Rosae Chinensis, 12 g
Radix Angelicae Sinensis, 30 g
Radix Salviae Filtiorrhizae, 30 g
crystal sugar, 50 g
millet wine, 1000 ml

**Process** Cut the first three ingredients into pieces and soak them in millet wine, seal the container and put it in a cool and dark place for 7 days. Remove the dregs and mix dissolved crystal sugar with the extracts equally.

**Directions** Take 15 ml twice daily.

**Indications** Irregular menstrual cycles, dysmenorrhea, scanty menses with clots, amenorrhea.

### Recipe 15
**Ingredients**
Angelicae, 24 g
Fructus Evodiae, 24 g
Rhizoma Chuanxiong, 24 g
Radix Paeoniae Alba, 18 g
Poria, 18 g
Pericarpium Citri Reticulatae, 18 g

Cortex Moutan Radicis, 18 g

Rhizoma Cyperi, 36 g

Radix Rehmanniae Praeparata, 36 g

Fructus Foenicuii, 12 g

Fructus Amomi, 12 g

plain spirits, 2500 ml

**Process**  Pound the above ingredients except plain spirits into pieces, fill them in a gauze bag and soak it in plain spirits in a pot, cover its lid, steam it in boiling water for two hours. The decoction can be taken 24 hours after it cools.

**Directions**  Take 20 ml twice daily.

**Indications**  Irregular menstrual cycles, distending pain in the lower abdomen. Contraindicated for cases with preceded menstrual cycles due to heat evil in the blood manifested by preceded menses accompanied with constipation and dark urine.

Recipe 16
**Ingredients**
Radix Angelicae Sinensis, 15 g

Rhizoma Corydalis, 15 g

Radix Achyranthis Bidentatae, 15 g

Flos Carthami, 15 g

Radix Curcumae, 15 g

plain spirits, 250 ml

**Process**  Cut the first five ingredients into pieces and soak them in plain spirits, seal the container and put it in a cool, dark place for 15 days.

**Directions**  Take 10 ml twice daily. Start the treatment two days prior to the coming menstruation. One course consisting of four months' treatment.

**Indications**  Menstrual period of over 7 days, metrostaxis, dysmenorrhea.

Recipe 17
**Ingredients**
Fructus Lycii, 60 g

Cortex Eucommiae, 250 ml

**Process**  Soak wolfberry fruit and eucommia bark in plain spirits and seal the container for 3 to 5 days. Filter the tincture and store the extracts up for future use.

**Directions**  Take 10 ml twice daily.

**Indications**  Irregular menstrual cycles, scanty menses of light red color, accompanied by dusty complexion, dizziness, tinnitus, soreness of the waist and knees, dull pain in the lower abdomen, nocturia, loose stools.

**Recipe** 18
**Ingredients**
Herba Serissae, 25 g
pork, 100 g
millet wine, 10 ml

**Process**  Cook pork with serissa (to be washed clean first) in a right amount of water for one hour. Condiments can be added according to one's taste. After it is done, add 10 ml of millet wine in the soup.

**Directions**  Take the meat and soup once daily.

**Indication**  Scanty menses.

**Recipe** 19
**Ingredients**
Receptaculum Nelumbinis, 100 g
millet wine, right amount

**Process**  Parch lotus receptacles with their nature retained. Grind the parched receptacles into fine powder and store up for later use.

**Directions**  Take 10 g of the powder with warm millet wine.

**Indication**  Menorrhagia.

**Recipe** 20
**Ingredients**
Herba Leonuri, 25 g
Herba Lycopi, 15 g
white sugar, 50 g
plain spirits, 100 ml

**Process**  Decoct the first three ingredients in 100 ml of plain spirits and 100 ml of water until 100 ml of the decoction retained.

**Directions**  Take 50 ml of the decoction twice daily.

**Indication**  Scanty menses.

**Recipe** 21
**Ingredients**
Rhizoma Nelumbinis Recens, 100 g
Cacumen Platycladi Orientalis, 60 g
millet wine, right amount

**Process**  Pound the first two ingredients into mash to extract juice for future use.

**Directions**  Take one half of the juice with warm millet wine, twice daily.

**Indication**  Amenorrhea.

**Recipe** 22
**Ingredients**
Radix Angelicae Sinensis, 30 g
Radix Codonopsis Pilosulae, 20 g
rice wine, 500 ml

**Process**  Soak the first two ingredients in rice wine and seal the container for over 7 days. Remove the dregs and store the tincture up for future use.

**Directions**  Take 30 ml twice daily. The treatment starts after the menstruation. One course consisting of six to seven days.

**Indication**  Delayed menstrual cycles due to deficiency of blood.

**Recipe** 23
**Ingredients**
Herba Allii Tuberosi, 250 g
rice wine, 60 ml

**Process**  Make decoction with Chinese chives in a right amount of water.

**Directions**  Take the decoction with rice wine, once daily. One course consisting of 5 days.

**Indication**  Menorrhagia due to deficiency of qi.

**Recipe** 24
**Ingredients**
Cyprinus Carpio, 1 (about 500 g)
millet wine, 250 ml

**Process**  Remove the scales and internal organs of the fish, wash it clean and cut into thin slices. Cook the fish in millet wine until they are done. Bake the bones of the fish to dry and grind them into fine powder.

**Directions**  Take the fish and powder with warm a right amount of millet wine before breakfast, daily.

**Indications**  Menorrhagia, menstrual period of over 10 days.

## Section 2  Dysmenorrhea

Dysmenorrhea refers to the periodic pain, intolerable in severe case, involving the lower abdomen or affecting the lumbosacral region prior to, post or during the menstrual flow. It is mostly complained of by young women.

The etiology of dysmenorrhea concerns with the impaired circulation of qi and blood due to either the deficiency of qi and blood or stagnation of qi and blood, leading to the disharmony between the Chong and Ren Channels and blood stasis in the uterus in the consequence of dysmenorrhea.

The excess type: The onset is caused by cold-damp retention in the Chong and Ren Channels, and blood stasis in the uterus due to factors such as catching cold, intake of cold food or dwelling in damp places during the menstrual period. Liver qi stagnation with subsequent stagnant qi and blood stasis may also impede the normal menstrual flow and develop dysmenorrhea by means of obstruction.

The deficiency type: Deficiency of the liver and kidney, grand multiparity, or surviving some prolonged illness can cause the deficiency of both qi and blood, insufficiency of the Chong Channel and poor nourishment of uterine collaterals, leading to the pain during menstrual flow.

### Recipe 1
**Ingredients**
Radix Angelicae Sinensis, 250 g
plain spirits, 1000 ml
**Process**   Cut Chinese angelica into thin slices, soak them in plain spirits, seal the container for 3 to 5 days.
**Directions**   Take 10 ml three times daily.
**Indications**   Dysmenorrhea, constipation, postpartum pain in the lower abdomen due to blood stasis obstructing the collaterals.

### Recipe 2
**Ingredients**
Flos Carthami, 200 g
brown sugar, 20 g
plain spirits, 1000 ml
**Process**   Wash safflower clean, dry them in the sun, fill them along with brown sugar in a gauze bag, soak it in plain spirits, seal the container for 7 days.
**Directions**   Take 20 ml once daily.
**Indications**   Dysmenorrhea due to deficiency of blood or blood stasis.

### Recipe 3
**Ingredients**
Pericarpium Zanthoxyli, 1 g
plain spirits, 5 ml
**Process**   Grind bunge pricklyash peel into powder.
**Directions**   Take the powder with warm plain spirits.
**Indication**   Dysmenorrhea.

### Recipe 4
**Ingredients**

salt, 250 g

plain spirits, right amount

**Process**   Stir-fry salt with a right amount of plain spirits until it is hot enough to take effects.

**Directions**   Fill the salt in a gauze bag, apply it on the patient's umbilicus and lower abdomen for 30 minutes, three times daily. The salt be reheated several times during the course of treatment. One course consisting of 3 days.

**Indication**   Dysmenorrhea due to stagnation of qi and blood stasis.

**Recipe 5**

**Ingredients**

Rhizoma Chuanxiong, 5 g

egg, 2

millet wine, 20 ml

**Process**   Decoct Szechuan lovage rhizome and eggs in a right amount of water until they are done. Remove the dregs and eggshells, add millet wine in the decoction.

**Directions**   Take the eggs and the decoction once daily. One course consisting of seven days.

**Indication**   Dysmenorrhea.

**Recipe 6**

**Ingredients**

crab, 2 (about 250 g)

Rhizoma Homalomenae, 30 g

rice wine, 50 ml

**Process**   Cook crabs with homalomena rhizomes in a right amount of water over a slow fire until they are done. Add in rice wine and keep on cooking for a few minutes. Take the pot away from the fire, remove the dregs.

**Directions**   Take the crabs along with the soup, once daily.

**Indication**   Dysmenorrhea due to stagnation of qi and blood stasis.

## Section 3   Amenorrhea

Amenorrhea refers to any female who does not experience the first menstrual flow at the of 18, or an adult woman who ceased to have menstrual flow over a period of more than three months. The former is called the primary amenorrhea while the latter the secondary amenorrhea. It is clinically divided into deficiency and excess types. The former is related to deficiency of blood in which there is no flow to be released because of the emptiness of the Chong and Ren Channels. The latter is due to the obstruction of the Chong and Ren Channels by stagnation of qi and stasis of blood which blocks the menstrual flow. Specifically, over consumption of blood due to deficiency of the liver and kidney, chronic illness with weak constitution, or poor nourishment of the Chong and Ren Channels due to deficiency of the spleen and stomach and subsequent insufficiency of the acquired energy, can both lead to the deficient type of amenorrhea. Emotional disturbances with subsequent disorderly qi mechanism, or retention of pathogenic wind-cold and over intake of cold or raw food can both cause the blockage of qi and blood of the Chong and Ren Channels, resulting in excess type of amenorrhea.

### Recipe 1
**Ingredients**
Flos Rosae Chinensis, 15 g
Herba Leonuri, 15 g
millet wine, right amount
**Process**  Make decoction with the first two ingredients in a right amount of water.
**Directions**  Take the decoction with a right amount of millet wine.
**Indication**  Amenorrhea.

### Recipe 2
**Ingredients**
Semen Sinapis Albae, 60 g
millet wine, right amount
**Process**  Grind white mustard seeds into fine powder and store up for future use.
**Directions**  Take 6 g with warm millet wine before meals.
**Indications**  Amenorrhea accompanied with abdominal pain.

### Recipe 3
**Ingredients**
egg, 2
Rhizoma Curcumae Longae, 21 g
millet wine, right amount
**Process**  Cook eggs in water until they are done. Remove the eggshells and keep on cooking with fresh turmeria rhizomes for 20 minutes.
**Directions**  Take the eggs with warm millet wine, once daily. One course consisting of 5 days.
**Indication**  Amenorrhea.

### Recipe 4
**Ingredients**
Retinervus Luffae Fructus, 30 g
plain spirits, right amount
**Process**  Burn vegetable sponges into charcoal and grind it into powder.

**Directions**　　Take 9 g with plain spirits, once daily.
**Indication**　　Amenorrhea.

**Recipe** 5
**Ingredients**
Semen Juglandis, 9 g
Semen Oryzae cum Monasco, 12 g
millet wine, 60 ml
**Process**　　Stir-fry the first two ingredients in a right amount of vegetable oil until they are done.
**Directions**　　Take them with warm millet wine, once daily. One course consisting of 5 days.
**Indication**　　Amenorrhea.

**Recipe** 6
**Ingredients**
Auricularia, 30 g
Lignum Sappan, 30 g
plain spirits, 60 ml
**Process**　　Decoct the first two ingredients in 600 ml of water over a slow fire until 300 ml of decoction retained. Remove sappan wood from the decoction.
**Directions**　　Take the decoction and fungi once daily.
**Indication**　　Amenorrhea accompanied by distention of the waist and abdomen.

## Section 4　Metrorrhagia

Metrorrhagia refers to the type of uterine bleeding irrelevant to the normal menses. In traditional Chinese medicine, metrorrhagia is divided into the profuse and dripping ones. The former is characterized by a sudden onset of massive bleeding while the latter by a gradual dripping of blood from the uterus, occurring alternately. It is one of the common gynecological conditions, pertaining to dysfunctional uterine bleeding in modern medicine, and more complained of by women in their adolescence and climacterium. The chief cause of metrorrhagia is concerned with the impairment of the Chong and Ren Channels that fails to restrict the blood in the uterus. Such an impairment is often due to the damage of the spleen by over worry with subsequent deficiency of qi of the middle jiao that is unable to control the blood, or due to deficiency of kidney qi. Besides, invasion of exogenous pathogenic heat, or emotional disturbance with stagnation of liver qi turning into fire can both cause retention of heat in the lower jiao forcing the blood to flow outside of the normal channel.

### Recipe 1
**Ingredients**
chicken's liver, one set
rice wine, 200 ml
**Process**   Pound the liver into mash, cook it in rice wine until 100 ml of the soup retained.
**Directions**   Take one half of the liver and soup warmly, twice daily.
**Indication**   Metrorrhagia due to deficiency of kidney qi.

### Recipe 2
**Ingredients**
Crinis Carbonisatus, 90 g
millet wine, right amount
**Process**   Grind carbonized hair into powder.
**Directions**   Take 9 g of the powder with warm millet wine.
**Indications**   Metrorrhagia and metrostaxis.

### Recipe 3
**Ingredients**
Semen Sojae Nigrum, 60 g
egg, 2
millet wine, 120 ml
**Process**   Cook the eggs until they are done. Remove the shells of the eggs and recook them with black soya beans in 200 ml of water over a slow fire. After they have been done, add 120 ml of millet wine in the soup.
**Directions**   Take the eggs and black soya beans along with the soup, once daily.
**Indications**   Menorrhagia, delayed menstrual cycle of asthenic-cold type.

### Recipe 4
**Ingredients**
old hen, 1
Folium Artemisiae Argyi, 15 g
rice wine, 60 ml
**Process**   Remove the feathers and internal organs of the hen, wash it clean, cook it with argyi leaves and rice wine in a right amount of water. Condiments may be added according to one's taste.
**Directions**   Take all the meat and soup within two days. One course consisting of two weeks.
**Indications**   Metrorrhagia or metrostaxis, general weakness.

### Recipe 5
**Ingredients**
egg, 3

vinegar, 100 ml

millet wine, 100 ml

**Process**  Remove the shells of the eggs, Cook them in vinegar and millet wine until 100 ml of the soup retained.

**Directions**  Take 50 ml of the soup warmly before meals, twice daily.

**Indications**  Metrorrhagia and metrostaxis.

**Recipe** 6

**Ingredients**

cock, 1 (500 g)

rice wine, 100 ml

**Process**  Kill the cock to get blood. Put the blood in rice wine and stir the mixture well.

**Directions**  Take all the mixture within one day.

**Indications**  Metrorrhagia over a long period of time manifested by profuse uterine bleeding, dizziness, pallor.

**Recipe** 7

**Ingredients**

egg, 1

Succus Nelumbinis Recens, 20 ml

Radix Notoginseng, 3 g

old millet wine, 5 ml

**Process**  Grind notoginseng into powder, remove the shell of the egg, mix the ingredients equally in a pot. Cook the pot in boiling water until the mixture is done.

**Directions**  Take the mixture including the soup once or twice daily.

**Indications**  Dysfunctional uterine bleeding.

## Section 5  Abnormal Leukorrhea

Leukorrhea refers to abnormal vaginal discharge of an abnormal color, quality and odor. It is often due to over thinking, impairment of the spleen and stomach with subsequent poor transforming and transporting and retention of dampness and water which flow downward to the lower jiao, or due to over sexual indulgence, multiple labor with subsequent deficiency of kidney qi and vital essence, leading to the poor restriction of the Dai Channel. It may also be caused by the downward flow of damp-heat along the Liver Meridian of Foot-Jueyin to the lower jiao.

### Recipe 1
**Ingredients**

Colla Plastri Testudinis, 10 g

millet wine, 50 ml

**Process** Make decoction with tortoise-plastron glue in millet wine until it dissolves.

**Directions** Take the decoction before breakfast, daily. One course consisting of 5 to 7 days.

**Indications** Profuse leucorrhea, leukorrhea with bloody discharge. Contraindicated for cases with distention of the abdomen and loose stools due to deficiency of spleen yang.

### Recipe 2
**Ingredients**

Cortex Lycii Radicis, 90 g

Rhizoma Dioscoreae, 50 g

Cortex Eucommiae, 50

plain spirits, 1000 ml

**Process** Mix hypoglauca yams and eucommia bark with honey and stir-fry them in an earthenware pot until they are done. Pound and grind the first three ingredients into fine powder, soak it in plain spirits in an earthenware pot, cover the lid, cook the pot in boiling water for over one hour. After it cools, filter the decoction and store the extracts up in a clean bottle for later use.

**Directions** Take 10 ml three times daily.

**Indications** Leukorrhagia, lumbago, frequency of micturition.

### Recipe 3
**Ingredients**

Carapax Trionycis, 9 g

plain spirits, right amount

**Process** Bake tortoise shell until it becomes brown, grind it into fine powder.

**Directions** Take 9 g of the powder with warm millet wine, once daily.

**Indications** Leucorrhagia accompanied with distending pain in the lumbar region due to impairment of kidney qi.

### Recipe 4
**Ingredients**

Semen Benincasae, 200 g

millet wine, 500 ml

**Process** Bake waxgourd seed until they become yellowish, grind them into powder, soak in millet wine, seal the container for 10 days.

**Directions** Take 15 ml twice daily.

**Indication** Leukorrhagia due to deficiency of kidney qi.

**Recipe** 5

**Ingredients**

Herba Portulacae, 300 g

millet wine, 500 ml

**Process** Remove the root and wash portulaca clean, pound into mash, soak it in millet wine, seal the container for 3 days. Then filter the tincture with a piece of gauze, store the extracts up in a clean bottle for future use.

**Directions** Take 15 ml twice daily.

**Indications** Leukorrhagia of yellow color, renal tuberculosis.

**Recipe** 6

**Ingredients**

Semen Apium, 50 g

millet wine, 500 ml

**Process** Soak the seed in millet wine, seal the container for 5 days. Store the tincture up for future use.

**Directions** Take 15 ml once or twice daily.

**Indications** Leukorrhagia, postpartum epigastric pain due to attacking of cold evil.

**Recipe** 7

**Ingredients**

Fructus Rosae Laevigatae, 120 g

Fructus Euryales, 120 g

rice wine, 1000 ml

**Process** Wash cherokee rose-hip clean and pound into pieces, grind dried fruit of gordon euryale into powder. soak the ingredients in rice wine and seal the container for 5 to 7 days. Shake the container frequently during soaking. 5 or 7 days later, add 1 g of salt in the container, cover the lid, steam it in boiling water for 2 hours. After it cools, remove the dregs by filtering with a piece of gauze and store the extracts up for later use.

**Directions** Take 50 ml before meals, twice daily.

**Indication** Leukorrhagia.

**Recipe** 8

**Ingredients**

Flos Celosiae Cristatae, 180 g

rice wine, 1000 ml

**Process** Dry cockscomb flower in the sun and then grind into powder, soak in rice wine and seal the container for 5 to 7 days. Then filter the tincture and store the extracts up in a clean bottle for later use.

**Directions** Take 30 to 50 ml before breakfast, once daily.

**Indications**   Leukorrhagia, diarrhea.

**Recipe** 9
**Ingredients**
Semen Gossypii, 60 g
millet wine, right amount
**Process**   Stir-fry cotton seeds until they are done, grind them into fine powder.
**Directions**   Take 6 g of the powder with warm millet wine before meals, twice daily.
**Indication**   Leukorrhagia.

**Recipe** 10
**Ingredients**
Folium Artemisiae Argyi, 20 g
egg, 1
spirits, right amount
**Process**   Cook the egg with argyi leaves in spirits until it is done.
**Directions**   Take the egg once daily.
**Indication**   Leukorrhagia.

**Recipe** 11
**Ingredients**
Semen Allii Tuberosi
vinegar
millet wine
**Process**   Cook Chinese chive seeds in a right amount of vinegar until they are done. Bake them to dry and grind into powder. Mix it with honey to make pills the size of a red phaseolus bean.
**Directions**   Take 30 pills with warm millet wine before meals, twice daily. One course consisting of 7 to 8 days.
**Indication**   Leukorrhagia.

## Section 6   Infertility

A married woman who fails to become pregnant in two consecutive years of time, while the reproductive function of her marriage partner is medically proved normal, is considered to suffer from infertility. In traditional Chinese medicine, it is regarded to be concerned with congenital deficiency of kidney qi or insufficiency of essence and blood, leading to the deficiency of Chong and Ren Channels and malnutrition of the uterus with consequent infertility. On the other hand, the invasion of exogenous pathogenic cold retained in the uterus may cause stagnation of cold and blood stasis as well as the obstruction of the uterine collaterals. Moreover, poor function of the spleen in transporting and transforming as well as the habitual diet of oily greasy food brings on retention of phlegm-damp in the interior, leading to the impaired qi mechanism and obstruction of the uterine collaterals. Obstruction is thus the main barrier for pregnancy. The following prescriptions are effective for it in variable degrees.

### Recipe 1
**Ingredients**
Radix Camelliae Sinensis, 15 g
Radix Campsis, 30 g
hen, 1
brown sugar, right amount
millet wine, right amount
rice wine, right amount

**Process**  Make decoction with the first two ingredients in a right amount of millet wine in a pot (put the pot in boiling water) for two to three hours. Remove the dregs and add in brown sugar and store the decoction up for future use. Remove the feathers and internal organs of the old hen and cook it with the other ingredients (including the root of Chinese trumpetcreeper and the root of tea tree) until it is done. Salt and other condiments can be added according to one's taste.

**Directions**  Take the decoction one day before the coming menstruation. Take the hen one day after menstruation. One course consisting of three months.

**Indications**  Infertility accompanied with dysmenorrhea.

### Recipe 2
**Ingredients**
Herba Epimedii, 100 g
Herba Cistanchis, 50 g
rice wine, 1000 ml

**Process**  Soak the first two ingredients in rice wine and seal the container for 7 days. Remove the dregs and store the extracts up in a clean bottle for future use.

**Directions**  Take 10 ml before meals, three times daily.

**Indication**  Infertility due to deficiency of kidney yang.

### Recipe 3
**Ingredients**
Cornu Cervi Pantotrichum, 10 g
Rhizoma Dioscoreae, 30 g
millet wine, 500 ml

**Process**  Cut pilose antler and Chinese yams into thin slices, soak them in millet wine and seal the container for 7 days.

**Directions**  Take 10 ml before meals, three times daily.

**Indication**  Infertility due to deficiency of kidney yang.

## Section 7  Threatened Abortion

Threatened abortion refers to a syndrome comprises a group of symptoms and signs that are the indications of abortion, e.g., soreness of the waist, distending pain in the lower abdomen, or a small amount of vaginal bleeding during pregnancy. In traditional Chinese medicine, it is also known as "Taidongbu'an" or "Tailou". The latter refers to the single symptom of a small amount of vaginal bleeding. It is mainly due to incoordination between the Chong and Ren Channels in combination with disharmony between qi and blood circulation. Moreover, deficiency of both qi and blood can also lead to threatened abortion.

**Recipe** 1

**Ingredients**

Galla Chinensis, 15 g

millet wine, a right amount

**Process**  Grind Chinese gall into fine powder.

**Directions**  Take the powder with a right amount of warm millet wine, once daily.

**Indication**  Threatened abortion manifested by vaginal bleeding during pregnancy.

**Recipe** 2

**Ingredients**

Receptaculum Nelumbinis, 60 g

millet wine, a right amount

**Process**  Parch lotus receptacles into charcoal with their nature retained. Grind the parched receptacles into fine powder.

**Directions**  Take 6 g of the powder with a right amount of warm millet wine, once daily.

**Indication**  Threatened abortion manifested by vaginal bleeding during pregnancy.

**Recipe** 3

**Ingredients**

Rhizoma Atractylodis Macrocephalae, 60 g

millet wine, 50 ml

**Process**　Grind bighead atractylodes rhizome into fine powder. Decoct 6 g of the powder in 50 ml of millet wine until it has been brought to several times of boils.

**Directions**　Take the decoction warmly, once daily.

**Indication**　Threatened abortion due to deficiency of spleen qi.

### Recipe 4
**Ingredients**

Semen Sojae Nigrum, 60 g

millet wine, 30 ml

**Process**　Make decoction with black soya beans and millet wine in a right amount of water.

**Directions**　Take the decoction once daily.

**Indications**　Threatened abortion manifested by vaginal bleeding accompanied with abdominal pain and lumbago during pregnancy.

### Recipe 5
**Ingredients**

egg, 14

millet wine, 500 ml

**Process**　Mix the yolks of fourteen eggs with millet wine equally in a pot. Cook the mixture over a slow fire until it is done. After it cools, store up in a bottle for future administration.

**Directions**　Take 30 g of the mixture warmly, once daily.

**Indication**　Threatened abortion.

### Recipe 6
**Ingredients**

Radix Angelicae Sinensis, 25 g

Bulbus Allii, 15 g

millet wine, 20 ml

**Process**　Decoct Chinese angelica and Chinese green onion in 600 ml of water until 400 ml of decoction retained. Add in 20 ml of millet wine and keep on decocting until 300 ml of decoction left. Remove the dregs and store the decoction up for future administration.

**Directions**　Take 100 ml warmly, once daily.

**Indications**　Threatened abortion manifested by abdominal pain and lumbago during pregnancy.

### Recipe 7
**Ingredients**

Fructus Amomi, 100 g

millet wine, a right amount

**Process**　Bake amomum fruit to dry and grind them into fine powder.

**Directions**　Take 10 g of the powder with warm millet wine, once daily.

**Indications** Threatened abortion manifested by abdominal pain and lumbago during pregnancy.

## Section 8  Retention of Placenta

Retention of placenta refers to delayed relief of placenta 30 minutes after delivery. In traditional Chinese medicine, it is mostly due to weak constitution, deficiency of qi, prolonged labor course with over-consuming of both qi and blood. Invasion of pathogenic cold with consequent stagnation of qi and blood, and weakening of the uterine activity may also result in retention of placenta. The subsequent prescriptions are effective for this condition in variable degrees.

**Recipe** 1
**Ingredients**
Radix Angelica Sinensis, 9 g
Rhizoma Chuanxiong, 9 g
Semen Persicae, 9 g
Radix Glycyrrhizae Praeparata, 1.5 g
Radix Codonopsis Pilosulae, 9 g
Rhizoma Zingiberis Praeparata, 1.5 g
urine of a boy under 12, 10 ml
millet wine, 20 ml
**Process** Decoct the first six ingredients in urine and millet wine and a right amount of water.
**Directions** Take the decoction warmly.
**Indication** Retention of placenta.

**Recipe** 2
**Ingredients**
Faeces Trogopterorum, 5 g
Pollen Typhae, 5 g
millet wine, right amount
**Process** Grind the first two ingredients into fine powder.
**Directions** Take the powder with warm millet wine.
**Indication** Retention of placenta.

**Recipe** 3
**Ingredients**
egg, 1

millet wine, 20 ml

**Process**   Mix the shelled egg with millet wine equally.
**Directions**   Take the mixture warmly.
**Indication**   Retention of placenta.

**Recipe** 4
**Ingredients**
Semen Leonuri, 50 g

millet wine, 10 ml

**Process**   Pound motherwort fruit and to extract juice.
**Directions**   Take the juice with warm millet wine.
**Indication**   Retention of placenta.

**Recipe** 5
**Ingredients**
Semen Sojae Nigrum, 50 g

millet wine, 250 ml

**Process**   Make decoction with black soya beans in millet wine until 120 ml of decoction retained.
**Directions**   Take 40 ml of warm decoction three times within 2 hours.
**Indication**   Retention of placenta.

## Section 9   Postpartum Abdominal Pain

Postpartum abdominal pain, also known as puerperal pain, refers to the pain in the lower abdomen in puerperium. It is mostly complained by multipara and within 1-2 days after the delivery. It is also called baby pillow pain in TCM. According to traditional Chinese medicine, it is said to be concerned with heavy loss of blood during labour with subsequent emptiness of the Chong and Ren Channels causes malnutrition of the uterine collaterals or deficiency of both qi and blood, resulting in poor blood circulation and stagnant pain in the lower abdomen. The following prescriptions can alleviate the pain in various degrees.

**Recipe** 1
**Ingredients**
crab, 1

rice wine, 10 ml

**Process**  Wash the crab clean and stew it over a slow fire. When it is nearly done, add rice wine in and keep on stewing for a few minutes.

**Directions**  Take the flesh of crab along with the soup, once daily.

**Indications**  Postpartum abdominal pain, lochiostasis.

### Recipe 2
**Ingredients**
Fructus Evodiae, 12 g
Fructus Gardeniae, 10 g
Semen Persicae, 3 g
Flos Carthami, 3 g
Lignum Aquilariae Resinatum, 3 g
plain spirits, right amount

**Process**  Grind the first into fine powder.

**Directions**  Apply the powder with a right amount of plain spirits on the abdomen, and heat the points with moxa sticks for 10 minutes, once daily.

**Indication**  Postpartum abdominal pain.

### Recipe 3
**Ingredients**
Folium Camelliae Sinensis, 5 g
brown sugar, 50 g
millet wine, 10 ml

**Process**  Dissolve brown sugar in 50 ml of boiling water in a cup. Add tea in the cup and cover the lid for a few minutes.

**Directions**  Take the drink with millet wine warmly, once daily.

**Indications**  Postpartum abdominal pain, lochiorrhea.

### Recipe 4
**Ingredients**
Fructus Crataegi, 15 g
brown sugar, 50 g
rice wine, 10 ml

**Process**  Make decoction with the first two ingredients in a right amount of water.

**Directions**  Take the decoction with 10 of warm millet wine twice or three times daily.

**Indication**  Postpartum abdominal pain due to blood stasis resulting from cold-evil retention.

### Recipe 5
**Ingredients**
Fructus Crataegi, 50 g

Herba Leonuri, 50 g

millet wine, right amount

**Process**   Make decoction with the first two ingredients in a right amount of water. After the decoction has been done, remove the dregs for future use.

**Directions**   Take one third of the decoction with warm millet wine three times daily.

**Indication**   Postpartum abdominal pain.

### Recipe 6
**Ingredients**

mutton, 120 g

Radix Rehmanniae Praeparata, 60 g

Rhizoma Zingiberis, 60 g

millet wine, right amount

**Process**   Make decoction with the first three ingredients in a right amount of millet wine.

**Directions**   Take the decoction and mutton once daily.

**Indication**   Postpartum abdominal pain due to deficiency of blood resulting in cold-evil retention.

### Recipe 7
**Ingredients**

Resina Draconis, 5 g

Myrrha, 15 g

millet wine, right amount

**Process**   Grind the first two ingredients into fine powder.

**Directions**   Take the powder with warm millet wine.

**Indication**   Postpartum abdominal pain.

### Recipe 8
**Ingredients**

Herba Leonuri, 10 g

Radix Rehmanniae, 6 g

millet wine, 250 ml

**Process**   Put the above ingredients in an earthenware pot, cover its lid and steam the pot in boiling water for half one hour. Take out the pot and remove the dregs. Store the extracts in a bottle for future use.

**Directions**   Take 20 ml warmly, twice daily.

**Indications**   Postpartum abdominal pain, lochiorrhea.

# Section 10  Postpartum Hemorrhage

Postpartum hemorrhage refers to vaginal bleeding with the amounts of or over 400 ml twenty four hours after delivery. It is mainly due to uterine inertia. According to traditional Chinese medicine, this condition is due to impairment of qi and failure of the spleen to govern the circulation of blood.

**Recipe** 1
**Ingredients**
Radix Celosiae Cristatae, 30 g
millet wine, right amount
**Process**  Make decoction with the root of cockscomb flower in a right amount of millet wine.
**Directions**  Take the decoction warmly, once daily.
**Indication**  Postpartum hemorrhage.

**Recipe** 2
**The same as** Recipe 9 in Postpartum Abdominal Pain.
**Indication**  Postpartum hemorrhage.

**Recipe** 3
**Ingredients**
Cortex Trachycarpi, 90 g
millet wine, 5 ml
**Process**  Parch palmae bark with its nature retained, grind it into fine powder and store it up for future use.
**Directions**  Take 9 g with warm millet wine.
**Indication**  Postpartum hemorrhage.

**Recipe** 4
**Ingredients**
carp, Cyprinus Carpio, 1 (about 500 g)
millet wine, right amount
**Process**  Cut the fish open and remove its internal organs. Cook the carp in a right amount of millet wine.
**Directions**  Take the fish once daily. Bake the bones to dry and grind into powder, taken with millet wine before breakfast, daily.
**Indication**  Postpartum hemorrhage.

### Recipe 5
**Ingredients**
Rhizoma Corydalis, 30 g
millet wine, right amount

**Process**  Stir-fry corydalis tubers to dry and grind them into fine powder, store it up for future use.

**Directions**  Take 10 g with warm millet wine.

**Indications**  Postpartum hemorrhage, lochiorrhea accompanied with restlessness, feverish sensation in the palms and soles.

### Recipe 6
**Ingredients**
Semen Sojae Nigrum, 200 g
Semen Phaseoli, 200 g
millet wine, 20 ml

**Process**  Stir-fry black soya beans and red phaseolus beans until they are half-done. Make decoction with them in 20 ml of millet wine and a right amount of water.

**Directions**  Take the decoction once daily.

**Indications**  Postpartum hemorrhage, lochiorrhea.

### Recipe 7
**Ingredients**
Herba Cirsii Japonisi, 200 g
Herba Cephalanoploris, 200 g
millet wine, 600 ml

**Process**  Soak the first two ingredients in plain spirits and seal the container for 5 days. Remove the dregs and store the extracts up in a clean bottle for future use.

**Directions**  Take 20 ml warmly.

**Indications**  Postpartum hemorrhage, lochiorrhea, metrorrhagia.

### Recipe 8
**Ingredients**
Radix Codonopsis Pilosulae, 25 g
Radix Astragali, 25 g
Radix Angelicae Sinensis, 25 g
mutton, 500 g
millet wine, 50 ml

**Process**  Wash the meat clean and cut into cubes. Fill the first three ingredients in a gauze bag and fasten its mouth. Put the meat along with the bag in an earthenware pot. Add millet wine and a right amount of water in it and began to cook the meat over a strong fire until the water boils. Then keep on cooking over a slow fire until the mutton is completely done. Condiments are then added according to one's taste.

**Directions**  Take all the meat and soup within two days.

**Indication**  Postpartum hemorrhage due to deficiency of qi failing to control the circulation of blood.

**Recipe** 9
**Ingredients**
Radix Notoginseng, 3 g
Cortex Trachycarpi, 8 g
millet wine, right amount

**Process**  Parch palmae bark with its nature retained. Then grind it along with notoginseng into fine powder.

**Directions**  Take the powder with warm millet wine.

**Indication**  Postpartum hemorrhage.

**Recipe** 10
**Ingredients**
Rhizoma Anemones Altaicae, 20 g
Radix Sanguisorbae, 50 g
Radix Angelicae Sinensis, 40 g
millet wine, 500 m

**Process**  Grind the first three ingredients into fine powder. Make decoction with the powder in millet wine until it is done. Remove the dregs and store the extracts up for future use.

**Directions**  Take 10 ml warmly.

**Indication**  Postpartum hemorrhage.

**Recipe** 11
**Ingredients**
Radix Rehmanniae Praeparata, 50 g
Radix Angelicae Sinensis, 50 g
millet wine, 500 ml

**Process**  Pound and grind the first ingredients into fine powder. Make decoction with the powder in millet wine until it is brought to several times of boils. Remove the dregs and store the extracts up for future use.

**Directions**  Take 20 ml warmly, three times daily.

**Indication**  Postpartum hemorrhage accompanied with abdominal pain.

## Section 11  Lochiorrhea

Lochia refers to vaginal discharge of cellular debris, mucus and blood following childbirth. The complete discharge needs three weeks of time. Persistent vaginal discharge over three weeks after delivery is called lochiorrhea. The condition may be due to weak constitution with deficiency of antipathogenic qi, or over consumption of both qi and blood during delivery, early physical labor after childbirth which results in sinking of qi and poor consolidation of the Chong and Ren Channels so as to fail to govern the blood. Excessive loss of yin fluid with subsequent yin deficiency causes heat in the interior. Invasion of exogenous pathogenic heat or heat transformed from liver qi stagnation may all stay in the interior. Such factors may disturb the Chong and Ren Channels impending a disorderly blood circulation that develops into lochiorrhea. However, invasion of exogenous pathogenic cold encountering blood in the body may produce blood stasis in the uterus, which also results in the incoordination of the Chong and Ren Channels, and lochiorrhea occurs.

### Recipe 1
**Ingredients**
dried persimmon, 3
millet wine, right amount
**Process**  Burn dried persimmons into charcoal with their nature retained. Grind them into powder and store it up for future use.
**Directions**  Take 10 g of the powder with a right amount of warm millet wine.
**Indication**  Lochiorrhea.

### Recipe 2
**Ingredients**
Herba Serissae, 30 g
Radix Glycyrrhizae, 30 g
millet wine, right amount
**Process**  Pound and grind the first two ingredients into powder and stir it equally. Make decoction with 20 g of such powder in 50 ml of water. After it is done, remove the dregs and add in 10 ml of millet wine.
**Directions**  Take the decoction warmly.
**Indication**  Lochiorrhea due to postpartum blood stasis.

### Recipe 3
**Ingredients**
Semen Oryzae cum Monasco, 12 g

millet wine, 100 ml

**Process**  Make decoction with rice fermented with red yeast in millet wine. After it is done, remove the dregs for future use.

**Directions**  Take the decoction warmly.

**Indication**  Lochiorrhea.

**Recipe** 4
**Ingredients**
crab, 200 g

millet wine, 100 ml

**Process**  Place the crab and millet wine in an earthenware pot, cover its lid, steam the pot in boiling water until the crab is done. Condiments can be added according to one's taste.

**Directions**  Take the crab and soup once daily.

**Indication**  Lochiorrhea accompanied with stabbing pain in the lower abdomen.

## Section 12  Galactostasis

Galactostasis refers to retention of milk accompanied by other symptoms involve the breast. According to traditional Chinese medicine, this condition is due to stagnation of liver qi accompanied with exogenous pathogenic wind-heat.

**Recipe** 1
**Ingredients**
Folium Heleodaris, 30 g

plain spirits, right amount

**Process**  Cut fresh leaves of water chestnut into pieces, add in a right amount of plain spirits, pound them into mash. Stir-fry the mash until it is hot enough to take effects.

**Directions**  Apply the mash on breast(s) once daily.

**Indication**  Galactostasis.

**Recipe** 2
**Ingredients**
Fructus Luffae, 30 g

millet wine, right amount

**Process**  Burn luffa fruits into charcoal with their nature retained. Grind them into fine powder and store it up for future use.

**Directions**     Take 3 to 6 g with warm millet wine to get mild perspiration.
**Indication**     Galactostasis.

**Recipe 3**
**Ingredients**
Semen Citri Reticulatae, 15 g
rice wine, 30 ml
**Process**     Pound tangerine seeds into mash, decoct it in 30 ml of rice wine until 10 ml of decoction retained.
**Directions**     Take 10 ml of decoction twice daily.
**Indication**     Galactostasis accompanied with swelling pain in the breasts.

**Recipe 4**
**Ingredients**
Folium Chrysanthemi, 30 g
rice wine, right amount
**Process**     Pound chrysanthemum leaves into mash and extract it to get juice. Make decoction with the juice in 30 ml of rice wine until 15 ml of decoction retained.
**Directions**     Take 15 ml of the decoction warmly. Apply hot dregs on the affected part.
**Indication**     Distending pain in the breast due to obstruction of lactiferous ducts.

**Recipe 5**
**Ingredients**
Folium Chrysanthemi, 15 g
Pericarpium Citri Reticulatae Viride, 15 g
Cornu Cervi Degelatinatum, 15 g
millet wine, 10 ml
**Process**     Make decoction with the first three ingredients in a right amount of water. After it is done, remove the dregs, add 10 ml of millet wine in the decoction.
**Directions**     Take the decoction warmly.
**Indication**     Galactostasis.

**Recipe 6**
**Ingredients**
Folium Carotae
plain spirits
**Process**     Extract a right amount of fresh carrot leaves to get 10 ml of juice.
**Directions**     Take the juice with 5 ml of warm plain spirits.
**Indications**     Galactostasis accompanied with swelling pain in the breast(s).

**Recipe** 7
**Ingredients**
Cornu Cervi, 10 g
millet wine, 10 ml
**Process**  Cut deer horn into thin slices, stir-fry them and grind them into fine powder.
**Directions**  Take the powder with warm millet wine, twice daily.
**Indications**  Galactostasis accompanied with distending pain in the breast(s).

**Recipe** 8
**Ingredients**
Semen Vaccariae, 10 g
Radix Trichosanthis, 10 g
Squama Manitis, 5 g
Radix Glycyrrhizae, 10 g
millet wine, right amount
**Process**  Bake pangolin scales until they become brown. Grind the first four ingredients into fine powder and store it up for future use. Make decoction with 7 g of the powder in 60 ml of millet wine until 30 ml of the decoction retained.
**Directions**  Take the decoction warmly, twice daily.
**Indication**  Galactostasis.

## Section 13  Hypogalactia

Hypogalactia, also known as lactation deficiency, refers to low or no production of milk after childbirth. Traditional Chinese medicine holds the view that milk is transformed from qi and blood. Either constitutional deficiency of spleen and stomach with insufficiency of the source of acquired energy, or heavy loss of blood which can not manufacture enough milk. Emotional depression after delivery may cause the liver to lose its maintenance over the free flow of qi with subsequent impairment of qi mechanism and obstructed qi circulation, leading to halted milk production.

**Recipe** 1
**Ingredients**
Semen Arachidis, 60 g
brown sugar, 30 g
millet wine, 30 ml
**Process**  Cook shelled peanuts in water until they are done. Add in brown sugar and millet wine

and keep on decocting them for a few minutes.

**Directions**   Take the peanuts and decoction, once daily.

**Indications**   Hypogalactia, galactostasis.

### Recipe 2
**Ingredients**
bean curd, 150 g
brown sugar, 50 g
rice wine, right amount

**Process**   Make decoction with the first two ingredients in a right amount of water. After brown sugar has dissolved, add rice wine in the decoction.

**Directions**   Take the decoction along with the dregs, once daily. One course consisting of 5 days.

**Indication**   Lack of lactation.

### Recipe 3
**Ingredients**
crab, 1
millet wine, 10 ml

**Process**   Pound the crab into mash, decoct it with 10 ml millet wine in a right amount of water.

**Directions**   Take the decoction and dregs, once daily.

**Indication**   Hypogalactia.

### Recipe 4
**Ingredients**
Carassius Auratus, 1 (about 500 g)
millet wine, 10 ml

**Process**   Remove the scales and internal organs of the fish, decoct it in a right amount of water until it is done. Add 10 ml of millet wine in the soup.

**Directions**   Take the fish and soup, once daily.

**Indication**   Hypogalactia.

### Recipe 5
**Ingredients**
Semen Sesami Nigrum, 15 g
rice wine, 10 ml

**Process**   Stir-fry black sesame seeds until they become brown, grind them into fine powder.

**Directions**   Take the powder with warm rice wine, once daily.

**Indication**   Hypogalactia.

**Recipe 6**
**Ingredients**
asparagus lettuce, 50 g
millet wine, 10 ml
**Process** Cut lettuces into small cubes and cook them in 200 ml of water until they are done. Add 10 ml of millet wine and small amount of salt in the soup.
**Directions** Take the lettuces and soup once daily.
**Indication** Hypogalactia.

**Recipe 7**
**Ingredients**
human placenta, one set
millet wine
**Process** Wash the placenta clean, bake it to dry and grind it into fine powder, store it up for future use.
**Directions** Take 4.5 g of the powder with 5 ml of millet wine, three times daily.
**Indication** Hypogalactia.

**Recipe 8**
**Ingredients**
lard, 20 g
white sugar, 10 g
egg, 2
rice wine, 200 ml
**Process** Cook the shelled eggs with cooked lard until they are half-done. Add rice wine in and keep on cooking until the eggs are completely done. Add white sugar in the cooked eggs.
**Directions** Take the eggs before breakfast, daily. One course consists of seven days.
**Indication** Hypogalactia.

**Recipe 9**
**Ingredients**
Macrobrachium Nipponense, 100 g
millet wine, 20 ml
**Process** Cut the feet of the shrimps off and decoct them in a right amount of water. After they have been done, add 20 ml of millet wine in the soup.
**Directions** Take the shrimps and soup, twice daily.
**Indication** Hypogalactia due to general weakness.

**Recipe** 10
**Ingredients**
pig trotter, 2
bean curd, 50 g
Bulbus Allii, 10 g
rice wine, 50 ml
soy sauce, 5 ml
**Process**  Cook the above ingredients in a right amount of water until they are done.
**Directions**  Take all the trotters and soup within one day.
**Indication**  Hypogalactia.

## Section 14  Prolapse of Uterus

Prolapse of uterus refers to different degrees of lapse of uterus, or even uterus lapsing out of the vaginal orifice in severe cases. It embraces the same prolapse of uterus and distention of vaginal wall in modern medicine. The main cause of prolapse of uterus, in traditional Chinese medicine, is considered to be concerned with deficiency of spleen qi and stomach qi and poor consolidation over uterus due to deficiency of kidney qi, both of which may lead to impairment of the uterine collaterals failing to keep the uterus in normal position. Over exhaustion of energy in delivery and early physical labor after delivery may cause deficiency and sinking of the spleen qi, which fails to do its normal heaving. Furthermore, multiple pregnancy and labors and over sexual indulgence with over consumptions of kidney qi can result in dysfunction of the Dai Channel in restricting and the incoordination between the Ren and Chong Channels, leading to prolapse of uterus. The following prescriptions are effective for this syndrome in variable degrees.

**Recipe** 1
**Ingredients**
Fructus Aurantii, 30 g
rice wine, 250 ml
**Process**  Cook citron fruit in rice wine over a slow fire.
**Directions**  Heat the pudendum by the steam of the decoction for 20 to 30 minutes.
**Indication**  Prolapse of uterus.

**Recipe** 2
**Ingredients**
Carassius Auratus, 250 g
rice wine, 100 ml
**Process**  Cook the head of crucian carp in rice wine along with a right amount of water to make

soup.

   **Directions**   Take the soup once daily.
   **Indication**   Prolapse of uterus.

**Recipe** 3
**Ingredients**
Carapax Trionycis, 180 g

millet wine, right amount

   **Process**   Parch the tortoise shells with their nature retained. Grind the parched shells into powder and store it up for future use.
   **Directions**   Take 6 g of the powder with a right amount of warm millet wine, three times daily.
   **Indication**   Prolapse of uterus.

**Recipe** 4
**Ingredients**
Retinervus Luffae Fructus, 30 g

plain spirits, 15 ml

   **Process**   Burn the first ingredient into charcoal and grind into powder and store it up for future use.
   **Directions**   Take 10 g of the powder with plain spirits, three times daily.
   **Indication**   Postpartum prolapse of uterus.

**Recipe** 5
**Ingredients**
Lumbricus, 7

millet wine, right amount

   **Process**   Bake earthworms to dry and grind them into fine powder.
   **Directions**   Take the powder with a right amount of warm millet wine, once daily.
   **Indication**   Prolapse of uterus.

**Recipe** 6
**Ingredients**
Fructus Litchi, 1000 g

rice wine, 1000 ml

   **Process**   Soak the shelled fruits in rice wine and seal the container for one week.
   **Directions**   Take 10 ml of the extracts twice daily.
   **Indication**   Prolapse of uterus.

# Section 15
# Other Proved Prescriptions For Postpartum Syndromes

**Recipe** 1
**Ingredients**
Flos Rosae Rugosae, 15 g
Radix Angelicae Sinensis, 60 g
Flos Carthami, 30 g
old rice wine, right amount
**Process**   Grind the first three dried ingredients into powder.
**Directions**   Take 3 g of the powder with warm rice wine, three times daily.
**Indications**   Paralysis, numbness of the limbs after delivery.

**Recipe** 2
**Ingredients**
Rhizoma Zingiberis, 1500 g
Fructus Jujubae, 250 g
Radix Allii Tuberosi, 200 g
rice wine, 500 ml
**Process**   Wash the first three ingredients clean and cut intopieces, put them in a pot and stir-fry them until they are half-done, add 500 ml of rice wine in and cover its lid for a few minutes.
**Directions**   Pick some dregs to make cakes the size of a coin and apply them on the affected areas for 10 hours daily. One course consisting of 5 days.
**Indications**   Contracture of the limbs after delivery, dyskinesia.

**Recipe**
**Ingredients**
Semen Sojae Nigrum, 500 g
plain spirits, 1000 ml
**Process**   Stir-fry black soya beans until they are half-done. Soak them in plain spirits and seal the container for 24 hours. Remove the beans and store the extracts up for future use.
**Directions**   Take 10 ml once daily.
**Indication**   Applied for postpartum health care.

**Recipe**
**Ingredients**
Arillus Longan, 500 g
plain spirits, 1000 ml

**Process**   Soak longan fruit in plain spirits and seal the container for over three months.

**Directions**   Take right amount of extracts after meals.

**Indications**   Edema, amnesia, palpitation, spontaneous perspiration, listlessness, anorexia after delivery.

**Recipe**

**Ingredients**

lard, 100 g

Succus Zingiberis, 100 g

millet wine, 50 ml

**Process**   Decoct the above ingredients in a pot until the decoction boils. After it cools, store it up in a bottle for future use.

**Directions**   Take one spoon of the extracts, dissolve it in boiling water for drinking, twice daily.

**Indication**   General weakness after delivery.

**Recipe**

**Ingredients**

egg, 2

rice wine, right amount

**Process**   Cook a right amount of rice wine until it boils. Add egg white in it and keep on cooking until the egg white is done.

**Directions**   Take the egg white once daily.

**Indication**   Applied for postpartum health care.

**Recipe**

**Ingredients**

Radix Astragali, 60 g

Radix Codonopsis Pilosulae, 30 g

Rhizoma Dioscoreae, 30 g

Fructus Jujubae, 30 g

hen, 1

millet wine, right amount

**Process**   Remove the feathers and internal organs of the hen, wash it clean, put it along with the first four ingredients in an earthenware pot. Add a right amount of millet wine in the pot to submerge the other ingredients. Cover the lid of the pot and steam it in boiling water until the hen is done.

**Directions**   Take the hen within two days.

**Indication**   For postpartum health care.

## Recipe 3
**Ingredients**

brown sugar, 100 g

millet wine, 150 ml

**Process**   Cook millet wine in a pot over a slow fire until it boils, add brown sugar in the pot and keep on cooking for a few minutes until 50 ml of the extracts retained.

**Directions**   Take the extracts once daily.

**Indication**   Postpartum diarrhea with no obvious causes.

## Recipe 4
**Ingredients**

Radix Ginseng, 15 g

plain spirits, 500 ml

**Process**   Soak ginseng in plain spirits and seal the container for 7 days.

**Directions**   Take 15 ml of the tincture once daily.

**Indication**   Pantalgia after delivery.

## Recipe 5
**Ingredients**

Cortex Acanthopanacis Radicis, 100 g

plain spirits, 500 ml

**Process**   Cut acanthopanax bark into pieces, soak them in plain spirits and seal the container for 7 days. Then filter the dregs out from the tincture and decoct 20 g of them in a right amount of water.

**Directions**   Take the decoction once daily.

**Indication**   Pantalgia after delivery.

## Recipe 6
**Ingredients**

Radix Angelicae Sinensis, 20 g

Rhizoma Chuanxiong, 6 g

Semen Persicae, 6 g

Radix Glycyrrhizae Praeparata, 3 g

Fructus Cannabis, 12

Pericarpium Citri Reticulatae, 10 g

plain spirits, 1 m

**Process**   Make decoction with the first six ingredients in water.

**Directions**   Take one half of the decoction with several drops of plain spirits, twice daily.

**Indication**   Postpartum constipation.

### Recipe 7
**Ingredients**
Radix Angelicae Sinensis, 50 g
Radix Rehmanniae Praeparata, 100 g
millet wine, right amount
**Process**  Make decoction with the first two ingredients in water.
**Directions**  Take the decoction with a right amount of millet wine, twice daily.
**Indication**  Postpartum fever due to deficiency of blood.

### Recipe 8
**Ingredients**
Pericarpium Citri Reticulatae, 50 g
millet wine, 10 ml
**Process**  Dry tangerine peel in the sun and then grind into powder.
**Directions**  Take 10 g of the powder with warm millet wine, once daily.
**Indication**  Postpartum paruria.

### Recipe 9
**Ingredients**
Flos Celosiae Cristatae, 15 g
plain spirits, 100 ml
**Process**  Make decoction with cockscomb flower in plain spirits.
**Directions**  Take the decoction once daily.
**Indication**  Pantalgia after delivery

### Recipe 10
**Ingredients**
Radix Astragali, 90 g
vinegar, 50 m
millet wine, 50 ml
**Process**  Make decoction with the above ingredients in a right amount of water.
**Directions**  Take the decoction warmly.
**Indication**  Postpartum faintness.

### Recipe 11
**Ingredients**
Herba Allii Tuberosi, 250 g
millet wine, 30 ml
**Process**  Cut Chinese chives into pieces and put them in a bowl. Decoct millet wine until it boils. Add boiling millet wine in the bowl and cover a lid for a few minutes to get extracts.

**Directions**  Take the extracts warmly.
**Indication**  Postpartum faintness.

**Recipe** 12
**Ingredients**
Cucumeris Sativus, 10 g
Pseudosciaena Polyactis, 10 g
urine of a boy under 12, 10 ml
millet wine, 10 ml
**Process**  Bake cucumber and air bladder of yellow croaker to dry and grind into fine powder.
**Directions**  Take the powder with urine and millet wine.
**Indication**  Postpartum faintness.

# Chapter Four  Pediatric Diseases

## Section 1  Hernia

An external hernia is an abnormal protrusion of intra-abdominal tissue or the whole or part of a viscus through an opening or fascial defect in the abdominal wall. A reducible hernia is one in which the contents of the sac return to the abdomen spontaneously or with manual pressure when the patient is recumbent. While an irreducible hernia is one whose contents cannot be returned to the abdomen, usually because they are trapped by a narrow neck. The definitive treatment of hernia is early operative repair. The subsequent prescriptions can improve the patient's symptoms in some degrees.

### Recipe 1
**Ingredients**
Semen Litchi, 100 g
millet wine, a right amount
**Process**  Stir-fry litchi seeds until they are done. Grind them into fine powder. Mix it with warm millet wine to make cakes the size of a coin.
**Directions**  Apply the warm cake on the affected part, twice or three times daily.
**Indication**  Infantile hernia manifested by pain and distention of the lower abdomen.

### Recipe 2
**Ingredients**
Sulphur, 9 g
Folium Artemisiae, 6 g
plain spirits, a right amount
**Process**  Fill a gauze bag with the first two ingredients, fasten the mouth, Decoct the bag in plain spirits until it boils.
**Directions**  Apply the hot bag on the affected part (the place where the patient complains of pains) for twenty to thirty minutes, three times daily. One course consisting of five days.
**Indication**  Hernia marked by pains due to cold retention resulting in stagnation of qi circulation.

## Section 2 Erysipelas

Erysipelas is an acute contagious skin condition marked by sudden onset of local redness, swelling, feverish sensation and pain. The lesion rises with clear-cut margins like scattered pieces of cloud. It is mostly caused by accumulation of damp-heat in the spleen and liver affecting the blood, or invasion of exogenous pathogenic wind-heat, dampness or fire in combination with deficiency of defensive qi.

**Recipe Ingredients**
Lumbricus, 30
Borneoli, 3 g
alcohol (75%), 60 ml

**Process**  Soak the first two ingredients in alcohol and seal the container for three days. Then store the tincture up for future administration.

**Directions**  Spread the tincture with a cotton swab over the affected areas, three times daily.

**Indication**  Erysipelas.

## Section 3 Eczema

Eczema is divided into two types: acute and chronic. The former is characterized by sudden onset of symmetric and polymorphic lesions in repeated attacks, and accompanied by erythema, edema, papule, vesiculation, oozing and intense itching. When cured, it presents decrustation without any traces. The latter is transformed from the acute eczema and characterized by roughness of skin, dark red or grey color of skin in the affected areas, scaled skin or lichen-like skin. Chronic eczema may often bring about acute attacks. The condition is mostly caused by invasion of exogenous pathogenic wind, heat and dampness at the superficial portion of the skin that halts the circulation of qi and blood and brings about obstruction of channels and collaterals, resulting in dormant damp-heat on the surface of the body. Moreover, dryness due to blood deficiency or malnutrition of the skin can also lead to chronic eczema.

**Recipe**
**Ingredients**
Alumen, a right amount
plain spirits, a right amount

**Process**  Parch alum until it is half-done. Grind it into fine powder.

**Directions** Spread a right amount of the powder with warm spirits on the affected part.
**Indication** Infantile eczema.

## Section 4 Enuresis

Enuresis refers to bed-wetting by children aged over three year old. It occurs several times at night for some severe cases. It is usually related to fatigue or mental stress. Bed-wetting due to excessive drinking of water on occasions is not considered as a morbid condition. Deficiency of kidney yang along with that of spleen qi and lung qi are the mains cause of enuresis.

**Recipe**
**Ingredients**
Rhizoma Zingiberis, 12 g
plain spirits, 100 ml
**Process** Pound ginger into mash and soak it in plain spirits, seal the container for three days.
**Directions** Spread a right amount of the tincture over the anterior mid-line inferior to the umbilicus with rubbing method until the skin becomes reddish. One course consisting of one week.
**Indication** Enuresis.

## Section 5 Vomiting

Recurrent vomiting may cause profuse loss of water and electrolytes leading to disturbance of metabolism. Inflammation of the respiratory tract or even asphyxia may occur when vomitus is inhaled into the lungs.

**Recipe 1**
**Ingredients**
Radix Rehmanniae, 9 g
rice wine, a right amount
**Process** Soak rehmannia root in rice wine for at least one hour.
**Directions** Spread the tincture over the soles of the patients, six times daily.
**Indication** Infantile vomiting.

**Recipe** 2
**Ingredients**
Rhizoma Zingiberis, 10 g
vinegar, 30 g
plain spirits, 30 ml
**Process**  Pound ginger into mash and mix it with the other ingredients equally.
**Directions**  Apply the mash on the soles of the patients, once daily.
**Indication**  Infantile vomiting.

## Section 6 Common Cold

Common cold is characterized by nasal obstruction and discharge, cough, headache, chills, fever and superficial pulse. It may occur around the year, but more often in autumn and winter. This condition embraces the upper respiratory tract inflammation due to viral or bacterial infection.

**Recipe** 1
**Ingredients**
Alumen, 12 g
flour, a right amount
plain spirits, a right amount
**Process**  Dissolve alum in plain spirits, mix a right amount of flour with the tincture to cakes the size of a coin.
**Directions**  Apply the cake on the soles of the patient, once or twice daily. One course consisting of three days.
**Indication**  Common cold manifesting wind-phlegm syndrome.

**Recipe** 2
**Ingredients**
Bulbus Heleodaris, 10
rice wine, 100 ml
**Process**  Cut water chestnuts into slices and cook them along with rice wine in a right amount of water until they are done.
**Directions**  Take the water chestnuts in order to cause mild perspiration.
**Indication**  Common cold.

## Section 7 Pertussis

Pertussis, also known as whooping cough, is one of the common respiratory infectious diseases suffered by infants. It is characterized by paroxysmal cough with spasm accompanied by a wheezing sound in the throat. Children mostly under the age of five may develop the condition all year round, especially in winter and spring. It is mostly caused by seasonal epidemic invasions that produce turbid phlegm in the interior, obstructing the passage of qi, which results in dysfunction of the lung to perform its normal dispersing and descending, the abnormal ascending of lung qi leads to this condition.

**Recipe**
**Ingredients**
Herba Ephedrae, 1.5 g
flour, 9 g
rice wine, a right amount
**Process**  Mix the above ingredients equally to make cakes the size of a coin.
**Directions**  Apply the cakes on Back-Shu Points on the back, twice or three times daily.
**Indication**  Whooping cough.

## Section 8 Varicella

Varicella is a contagious disease characterized by fever and a disseminated vesicular eruption. It is caused by the infection of varicella-zoster viruses.

**Recipe**
It is the same as **Recipe** 2 of Section 6.
**Indication**  Varicella.

# Chapter Five
# Diseases of Eyes, Ears, Nose and Throat

## Section 1 Conjunctivitis

Conjunctivitis, also known as "Hongyan" or "Huoyan" by Chinese convention, is characterized by redness and swelling in the palpebral, hyperemia of bulbar conjunctiva and profuse lacrimation, or even chemosis, corneal infiltration and corneal ulcer in severe cases. In traditional Chinese medicine, it is considered to be concerned with the invasion of wind-heat into the eye, or by ascending of sthenic fire in the liver and gallbladder. The following prescription is effective for conjunctivitis due to both exogenous invasion and internal fire.

**Recipe**
**Ingredients**
Radix et Rhizoma Rhei, 50 g
Semen Sojae Preparatum, 500 g
plain spirits, 1500 ml
**Process**   Grind rhubarb into fine powder. Fill it along with fermented soya beans in a gauze bag and fasten its mouth. Soak the bag in plain spirits and seal the container for 21 days.
**Directions**   Take 5 ml twice daily. One course consisting of 5 days.
**Indication**   Conjunctivitis.

## Section 2 Eye Injury

**Recipe**
**Ingredients**
Myrrha, 4.5 g
Resina Draconis, 4.5 g
Radix et Rhizoma Rhei, 9 g
Natrii Sulphas, 9 g
millet wine, right amount
**Process**   Grind the first four ingredients into fine powder.

**Directions**  Take the powder with a right amount of millet wine.
**Indication**  Applied for eye injury marked by hyphema as an accessory treatment.

## Section 3 Nyctalopia

Nyctalopia, also known as night blindness, is one kind of pathological change in the eyes caused by lack of vitamin A, which is also known as "Quemu" in traditional Chinese medicine. It is mainly due to insufficiency of both liver yin and kidney yin, manifested by gradual decrease in tears, dim vision at night or even being unable to see at all. Some cases may accompany with the symptoms and signs such as xerosis cutis, desquamation, pale tongue with little fur, thready and uneven pulse.

**Recipe 1**
**Ingredients**
Fructus Viticis, 500 g
plain spirits, 1000 ml
**Process**  Soak chastetree fruit in plain spirits and seal the container for 24 hours. Then put them in a pot, cover the lid, steam them for 20 minutes. Dry them in the sun and then grind into powder, mix it with honey equally to make pills. Each pill weighs 6 g.
**Directions**  Take one pill with rice water, twice daily.
**Indications**  Night blindness, optic atrophy, conjunctival congestion due to deficiency of liver yin.

**Recipe 2**
**Ingredients**
Semen Brassicae Rapae, 1000 g
plain spirits, a right amount
**Process**  Soak rutabaga seeds in plain spirits and seal the container for 24 hours. Then put them in a pot, cover the lid, steam the pot in boiling water for 20 minutes. Dry them in the sun and then grind into powder, mix it with honey equally to make pills. Each pill weighs 6 g.
**Directions**  Take one pill with rice wine, twice daily.
**Indication**  Night blindness.

**Recipe 3**
**Ingredients**
pork liver, 60 g
Bulbus Allii, 10 g

Rhizoma Zingiberis, 3 g

egg, 1

millet wine, a right amount

**Process**  Wash the liver clean and pound into mash. Cut Chinese green onion into pieces. Cook the green onion in a right amount of water and add in millet wine and powder of ginger in the mean time. When the soup boils, add the mash of pork liver and shelled egg in and keep on cooking for 5 minutes.

**Directions**  Take the soup along with the dregs, once daily.

**Indication**  Night blindness.

## Section 4 Diminution of Vision

**Recipe 1**

**Ingredients**

Fructus Mori, 5000 g

rice, 3000 g

distiller's yeast, a right amount

**Process**  Pound mulberries to extract their juice and cook it. Cook the rice until it is half-done. Mix the juice of mulberries and rice together in a pot, cover the lid and steam the pot until the rice is done. Add in a right amount of distiller's yeast and stir equally. Seal the pot and place it in a dry, cool place for a period of time until the extracts taste sweet. Then store the extracts up in a bottle for future use.

**Directions**  Take 20 ml with warm boiled water, twice daily.

**Indications**  Diminution of vision due to deficiency of liver yin and kidney yin.

**Recipe 2**

**Ingredients**

Fructus Lycii, 200 g

plain spirits, 300 ml

**Process**  Wash wolfberries clean and cut them into pieces, soak them in plain spirits and seal the container for 7 days. Shake the container once daily during soaking.

**Directions**  Take 10 to 20 ml of the extracts at bedtime, daily. After the extracts have been used up, take the dregs with a right amount of sugar.

**Indications**  Diminution of vision, irritated epiphora with tears due to deficiency of liver yin and kidney yin.

## Section 5 Pharyngitis

Pharyngitis is classified into two kinds: acute and chronic. The former manifests widespread red swelling in the throat, which also belongs to the category "Houbi" in traditional Chinese medicine; while the latter, also known as "Meiheqi" in traditional Chinese medicine, is a chronic and diffuse inflammation of the pharyngeal mucosa. Chronic pharyngitis is characterized by long-term discomfort, sensation of a foreign body or obstruction in the throat, itching, dryness, and mild soreness of the pharynx, coughing and vomiting may occur if the pharynx is further irritated. In traditional Chinese medicine, acute pharyngitis is due to invasion of exogenous pathogenic wind-heat attacking the Lung Meridian and Stomach Meridian resulting in heat accumulation in the throat, or constitutional heat accumulating in the lung and stomach flaring up to the throat; chronic pharyngitis is concerned with deficiency of kidney yin and over consumption of stomach yin resulting in the ascending of asthenic fire and lack of yin fluid to moisten the throat. The prescription here is effective for chronic cases.

**Recipe**
**Ingredients**
Radix et Rhizoma Rhei, 60 g
Mel, a right a mount
millet wine, a right amount
**Process**   Wash rhubarb clean and soak in millet wine for one hour, then put it in an earthenware pot, decoct it in 300 ml of water over a slow fire for 10 minutes. Filter the decoction to get the first extracts. Add 150 ml of water in the pot and keep on decocting the dregs for 10 minutes. Then remove the dregs and put the second extracts along with the first in another pot and cover the lid, steam the pot in boiling water for half one hour. After it cools, store the extracts up in a clean bottle for future use.
**Directions**   Take 10 ml with warm boiled water after meals, once to twice daily. Stop administration in case of the occurring of loose stools.
**Indication**   Chronic pharyngitis.

## Section 6 Acute Tonsillitis

Acute tonsillitis is an acute nonspecific inflammation of the palatal tonsillae. It is clinically manifested by fever, headache, sore throat which is aggravated in case of swallowing, and reddened and swollen palatal tonsillae. It is also known as "Ru'e" or "E'feng" in traditional Chinese medicine. It is caused by the attacking of wind-heat evil.

**Recipe**
**Ingredients**
Nidus Vespae, 30 g
millet wine, a right amount
**Process**  Bake the honey nest and grind it into fine powder.
**Directions**  Take 2 g of the powder with 20 ml of warm millet wine, every six hours.
**Indication**  Acute suppurative tonsillitis.

## Section 7 Aphonia

Aphonia is due to stagnation of qi and obstruction of the local collateral leading to failure of vocalizing.

**Recipe** 1
**Ingredients**
Semen Sinapis Albae, 150 g
plain spirits, 250 ml
**Process**  Fill a gauze bag with white mustard seeds and fasten the mouth of the bag. Soak it in plain spirits in an earthenware pot and start cooking over a slow fire until it boils.
**Directions**  Take 5 ml of the extracts orally twice to three times daily. Apply the hot bag on the neck and nape for 20 minutes, twice to four times daily. Reheat the bag during the treatment.
**Indications**  Aphonia due to sthenic cold evil in the lung, hoarseness due to edema of vocal cord.

**Recipe** 2
**Ingredients**
Lac Femininum, a right amount
millet wine, a right amount
**Process**  Mix human milk with millet wine equally.
**Directions**  Take a right amount of the mixture once daily.
**Indication**  Aphonia.

## Section 8  Paranasal Sinusitis

Paranasal sinusitis is divided into two kinds: acute and chronic. The former is manifested by stuffiness of nose, purulent nasal discharge, headache, fever, aversion to cold, anorexia, general discomfort, etc.. It is one of the commonly encountered nasal diseases in the clinic and results usually from acute rhinitis. It can be induced by general chronic diseases, malnutrition, lack of vitamins, drinking, smoking and catching cold. Acute paranasal sinusitis may develops into chronic type due to delayed treatment. Chronic paranasal sinusitis is characterized by nasal discharge of turbid substance, nasal obstruction and poor sense of smell, distending pain in the forehead and dizziness, hypomnesis. It is called "Biyuan" in traditional Chinese medicine. The condition is mainly due to invasion of exogenous pathogenic wind-cold evil attacking the superficial portion of the body and the lung. The wind-cold may transform into heat. The heat evil along with the poor function of the lung in descending and dispersing result in nasal obstruction and rhinorrhea with turbid discharge.

**Recipe**
**Ingredients**
Fructus Luffae, 150 g
millet wine, a right amount
**Process**   Bake the first ingredient and grind into powder.
**Directions**   Take 15 g of the powder with warm millet wine, twice daily.
**Indication**   Paranasal sinusitis.

## Section 9  Epistaxis

Epistaxis refers to nasal bleeding caused by factors other than traumatic injuries. It usually occurs on unilateral side and often on the anteroinferior part of the nasal septum. It can be caused by various of conditions. Long-term nosebleed may lead to secondary anemia.

**Recipe 1**
**Ingredients**
Concha Ostreae, 2 g
Gypsum Fibrosum, 1.5 g
plain spirits, 3 g
**Process**   Grind oyster shells and pypsum into fine powder and stir equally.
**Directions**   Take 3 g of the powder with plain spirits, three times daily.

**Indication**   Recurrent nosebleed.

**Recipe** 2
**Ingredients**
Bulbus Allii
plain spirits
**Process**   Pound a right amount of Chinese green onion into mash to get extracts.
**Directions**   Put the extracts with a right amount of plain spirits in the nasal cavity.
**Indication**   Epistaxis.

**Recipe** 3
It is the same as the prescription for conjunctivitis.
**Indication**   Epistaxis due to heat in the blood resulting in abnormal circulation.

**Recipe** 4
**Ingredients**
Napus
plain spirits
**Process**   Pound a right amount of radish to get 20 ml of extracts. Add in 1 ml of plain spirits and stir equally for use.
**Directions**   Take the extracts warmly.
**Indication**   Epistaxis.

## Section 10 Tympanitis

Tympanitis is characterized by otalgia, and purulent discharge from the ear. It is often caused by exogenous pathogenic wind-heat invasion into the ear along with the flaring-up of gallbladder fire and heat accumulation. Moreover, deficiency of spleen may also lead to tympanitis because poor function of spleen in transforming and transporting results in damp evil retention and turbid phlegm in the ear.

**Recipe** 1
**Ingredients**
Rhizoma Coptidis, 5 g
alcohol (75%), 25 ml
**Process**   Soak coptis root in the alcohol and seal the container for 3 days. Remove the dregs and store the tincture up for use.

**Directions**   Put a right amount of the tincture in the antrum auris, three times daily.
**Indication**   Chronic tympanitis.

### Recipe 2
**Ingredients**

Caulis Aristolochiae Manshuriensis, 5 g

Semen Strychni, 1 g

Fructus Evodiae, 2.5 g

rice wine, a right amount

**Process**   Grind the first three ingredients into powder and mix it with rice wine.
**Directions**   Put 5 drops of the mixture in the antrum auris, once every two hours. Five days consisting of one course.
**Indication**   Tympanitis.

## Section 11 Toothache

Toothache is commonly seen in the clinic. It can be caused by pulpitis, dental caries and periodontitis, and be aggravated by stimulation of either cold or heat. Toothache is due to invasion of exogenous pathogenic wind-fire obstructing the Yangming Meridian, which results in subsequent stagnation of qi and blood. Retention of heat in the stomach and intestine may also ascends to develop the condition. Furthermore, deficiency of kidney yin leads to the flaring up of asthenic fire which attacks the teeth.

### Recipe 1
**Ingredients**

Pericarpium Zanthoxyli, 7 grains

plain spirits, 100 ml

**Process**   Soak bunge pricklyash peel in plain spirits for future use.
**Directions**   Chew the pricklyash peel with the affected teeth.
**Indication**   Toothache.

### Recipe 2
**Ingredients**

Colophonium

plain spirits

**Process**   Grind colophony into fine powder and mix it with a right amount of plain spirits.

**Directions**　Apply the mixture on the gingivae.
**Indication**　Toothache.

### Recipe 3
**Ingredients**

Semen Juglandis, 50 g

plain spirits, 100 ml

**Process**　Cook the spirits until it boils. Soak walnut kernels in boiling spirits in a bowl covered with a lid.

**Directions**　Chew the walnut kernel slowly and then swallow it.

**Indication**　Toothache due to deficiency of kidney yin resulting in ascending of asthenic fire.

### Recipe 4
**Ingredients**

Semen Sojae Nigrum

millet wine

**Process**　Cook black soya beans in millet wine until the beans are done. Filter the decoction and store the extracts up for future use.

**Directions**　Gargle with the extracts.

**Indication**　Toothache, gingivitis.

# Chapter Six  Dermatoses

## Section 1 Urticaria

Urticaria, also known as wind wheal, refers to a sudden onset of skin eruption identified by red or white rash and itching sensation without any pain. The onset is often caused by wind invasion latent in the skin portion due to derangement of nutrient and defensive systems.

**Recipe** 1
**Ingredients**
Stigma Maydis, 15 g
rice wine, 100 ml
**Process**  Make decoction with corn stigmas in a right amount of water over a slow fire for twenty minutes, add in 100 ml of rice wine and keep on decocting until it is brought to boils.
**Directions**  Take the decoction once daily.
**Indication**  Urticaria.

**Recipe** 2
**Ingredients**
Herba Allii Tuberosi, 150 g
Bulbus Allii, 50 g
plain spirits, 30 ml
**Process**  Cut Chinese chives and Chinese green onion into thin slices, put them in an earthenware pot, add plain spirits and a right amount of water in, Make decoction over fire until it is done.
**Directions**  Take one half of the decoction, twice daily.
**Indication**  Urticaria.

**Recipe** 3
**Ingredients**
Radix Stemonae, 15 g
plain spirits, 100 ml
**Process**  Make decoction with tubers of stemona root in plain spirits.
**Directions**  Apply the decoction on the affected part with a piece of gauze three times daily.
**Indication**  Urticaria.

**Recipe 4**
**Ingredients**
Bombyx Batryticatus, 9 g
Periostracum Cicadae, 9 g
Radix et Rhizoma Rhei, 9 g
Rhizoma Curcumae Longae, 9 g
millet wine, a right amount
**Process**  Grind the first four ingredients into powder and store it up for administration.
**Directions**  Take 6 g with warm millet wine, twice daily.
**Indication**  Urticaria.

## Section 2 Psoriasis

Psoriasis refers to a chronic skin condition characterized by repeated sealed dermatosis which is difficult to be cured thoroughly. Some dry silver-white scales cover the affected areas and decrustate when scratching. Psoriasis is mostly caused by invasion of pathogenic wind, dampness and heat dormant between the skin and muscles. Furthermore, internal disturbance of wind and poor nourishment of skin resulting from deficiency of yin fluid and blood can also lead to roughness of skin, itching sensation and desquamation.

**Recipe 1**
**Ingredients**
Mylabris, 30
Pericarpium Citri Reticulatae Viride, 6 g
plain spirits, 250 ml
**Process**  Soak Chinese blistering beetles and green tangerine orange peel in plain spirits, seal the container and put it in a cool, dry place for seven days. Then filter the tincture and store it up for future administration.
**Directions**  Apply the tincture on the affected areas with a cotton swab with rubbing method until blisters occur. Stab the blisters with filiform needles in order to make them broken.
**Indication**  Psoriasis.

**Recipe 2**
**Ingredients**
Mylabris, 3
Radix Euphorbiae Kansui, 6 g
plain spirits, 100 ml

**Process** Soak the first two ingredients in plain spirits, seal the container and put it in a cool, dry place for seven days. Then filter the tincture and store it up for future administration.

**Directions** Apply the tincture on the affected areas with a cotton swab with rubbing method until blisters occur. Stab the blisters with filiform needles in order to make them broken.

**Indication** Psoriasis.

## Section 3 Frostbite

Frostbite refers to local pallor, cyanosis, itching, burning pain, edema, vesicles or even necrosis or ulceration on the local cutaneous lesions due to severe cold affection. It mostly occurs on hands, feet, facial region or auricles. It belongs to local chilblain in modern medicine. Frostbite is mainly caused by severe cold. It results in poor circulation of local qi and blood, leading to frostbite.

### Recipe 1
**Ingredients**
Pericarpium Zanthoxyli, 20 g
plain spirits, 200 ml

**Process** Soak bunge pricklyash peel in plain spirits, seal the container and put it in a cool, dry place for seven days. Then filter the tincture and store it up for future administration.

**Directions** Apply the tincture on the affected areas, once daily.

**Indication** Frostbite.

### Recipe 2
**Ingredients**
Semen Caryophylli, 15 g
plain spirits, 150 ml

**Process** Make decoction with cloves seeds in plain spirits until it boils.

**Directions** Apply the warm decoction on the affected areas, covered with a piece of gauze.

**Indication** Recurrent frostbite.

### Recipe 3
**Ingredients**
Rhizoma Zingiberis, 60 g
plain spirits, 100 ml

**Process** Soak ginger in warm plain spirits, seal the container for three hours. Then filter the tincture and store it up for future administration.

**Directions**   Apply the tincture on the affected areas, three times daily.
**Indication**   Primary frostbite.

## Section 4 Vitiligo

Vitiligo is a condition characterized by cutaneous patch of white color without subjective symptoms. It is mostly due to poor nourishment of the skin caused by derangement of qi and blood and stagnation of both qi and blood resulting from invasion of exogenous pathogenic wind into the skin portion.

**Recipe 1**
**Ingredients**
Fructus Mume, 50 g
Fructus Psoraleae, 60 g
plain spirits, a right amount
**Process**   Soak black plums and psoralea fruit in plain spirits, seal the container and put it in a cool, dry place for two weeks. Then filter the tincture and store it up for future administration.
**Directions**   Apply the tincture on the affected areas, three times daily.
**Indication**   Vitiligo.

**Recipe 2**
**Ingredients**
Receptaculum Fici Caricae, 20 g
plain spirits, 150 ml
**Process**   Wash the figs clean, cut them into thin pieces and soak them in plain spirits, seal the container and put it in a cool, dry place for seven days. Then filter the tincture and store it up for future administration.
**Directions**   Apply the tincture on the affected areas, three times daily.
**Indication**   Vitiligo.

**Recipe 3**
**Ingredients**
Herba Siegesbeckiae, 50 g
millet wine, a right amount
**Process**   Stir-fry siegesbeckia herbs with a right amount of millet wine until they are done. Bake them to dry and grind into fine powder, store it up for future administration.

**Directions**  Take 5 g of the powder with millet wine twice daily.
**Indication**  Vitiligo.

## Section 5  Alopecia

Alopecia refers to sudden regional loss of hair on the head. It is mostly caused by deficiency of liver and kidney with consequent failure of blood to nourish the hair. Invasion of wind evil in combination with deficiency of blood also leads to hair loss. Moreover, stagnation of liver qi may result in hair loss due to malnutrition due to stagnation of qi along with blood stasis.

**Recipe 1**
**Ingredients**
Rhizoma Drynariae, 15 g
Mylabris, 5
Radix Angelicae Dahuricae, 9 g
rice wine, 90 ml

**Process**  Soak the first three ingredients in rice wine, seal the container and put it in a cool, dry place for fifteen days. Then filter the tincture and store it up for future administration.

**Directions**  Apply the tincture on the affected areas, three to four times daily. One course consisting of 15 days.

**Indication**  Alopecia.

**Recipe 2**
**Ingredients**
beer, 150 ml

**Directions**  Apply beer on the hair and scalp, massage the scalp with one's hands for ten minutes, then have the hair washed with water.

**Indication**  Alopecia.

**Recipe 3**
**Ingredients**
Pericarpium Zanthoxyli, 120 g
alcohol, 500 ml

**Process**  Soak bunge pricklyash peel in alcohol, seal the container and put it in a cool, dry place for seven days. Then filter the tincture and store it up for future administration.

**Directions**  Apply the tincture on the affected areas, three times daily. One course consisting of

15 days.

**Indication**   Alopecia.

**Recipe** 4
**Ingredients**
Fructus Capsici, 10 g

plain spirits, 50 ml

**Process**   Soak hot peppers in plain spirits, seal the container and put it in a cool, dry place for ten days. Then filter the tincture and store it up for future administration.

**Directions**   Apply the tincture on the affected areas, several times daily.

**Indication**   Alopecia.

**Recipe** 5
**Ingredients**
Flos Sesami, 60 g

Flos Celosiae Cristatae, 60 g

plain spirits, 500 ml

**Process**   Cut the flowers into pieces and soak them in plain spirits, seal the container and put it in a cool, dry place for fifteen days. Then filter the tincture and add in 1.5 g of camphor, when it dissolves, store the tincture up for future administration.

**Directions**   Apply the tincture on the affected areas with a cotton swab, several times daily.

**Indication**   Alopecia.

## Section 6 Early Greying of Hair

Early greying of hair refers to the condition that the hair becomes white under 45 years. It is commonly seen in young Chinese and is mainly due to insufficiency of kidney yin and liver blood resulting in malnutrition of hair. However, Invasion of wind evil in combination with blood-heat can also lead to this condition.

**Recipe** 1
**Ingredients**
Radix Polygoni Multiflori, 40 g

Radix Rehmanniae, 40 g

plain spirits, 1000 ml

**Process**   Cut fleeceflower root into small cubes and rehmannia root into thin slices, soak them in plain spirits, seal the container and put it in a cool, dry place for fifteen days. Then filter the tincture and store it up for future administration.

**Directions**  Take 15 ml twice daily.

**Indications**  Early greying of hair accompanied with dizziness, lassitude, soreness of the loin and knees, emission, amnesia, insomnia, emaciation with sallow complexion due to deficiency of kidney yin and liver blood.

**Recipe** 2
**Ingredients**
Radix Polygoni Multiflori, 45 g
Radix Rehmanniae, 45 g
Radix Rehmanniae Praeparata, 45 g
Radix Asparagi, 45 g
Radix Ophiopogonis, 45 g
Fructus Lycii, 30 g
Radix Achyranthis Bidentatae, 30 g
Fructus Ligustri Lucidi, 30 g
Radix Angelicae Sinensis, 30 g
Semen Sojae Nigrum, 60 g
plain spirits, 2500 ml

**Process**  Pound the first ten ingredients into pieces and fill them in a gauze bag, fasten its mouth, soak it in plain spirits, seal the container and put it in a cool, dry place for fifteen days. Then filter the tincture and store it up for future administration.

**Directions**  Take 15 ml twice to three times daily.

**Indication**  Early greying of hair.

**Recipe** 3
**Ingredients**
Fructus Ligustri Lucidi, 80 g
Herba Ecliptae, 60 g
Fructus Mori, 60 g
millet wine, 1500 ml

**Process**  Pound the first two ingredients into pieces and mulberries into mash, fill them in millet wine, seal the container and put it in a cool, dry place for fourteen days. Shake the container several times during soaking. Then filter the tincture and store it up for future administration.

**Directions**  Take 20 ml warmly twice daily.

**Indications**  Early greying of hair, dizziness, soreness of the loin and knees, tinnitus due to deficiency of kidney and liver.

**Recipe** 4
**Ingredients**
Radix Cynanchi Auriculati, 250 g

Radix Polygoni Multiflori, 250 g

Radix Rehmanniae, 60 g

Fructus Jujubae, 45 g

Semen Juglandis, 45 g

Semen Nelumbinis, 45 g

Radix Angelicae Sinensis, 30 g

Fructus Lycii, 30 g

Radix Ophiopogonis, 15 g

Succus Zingiberis, 60 g

Mel, 45 g

rice wine, 3500 ml

**Process**  Pound the first nine ingredients into pieces, fill them in a gauze bag, fasten its mouth, soak it in plain spirits, add ginger juice in, seal the container and put it in a cool, dry place for fourteen days. Then filter the tincture and add honey in, stir the mixture equally, store it up for future administration.

**Directions**  Take 15 ml twice daily.

**Indications**  Early greying of hair, dizziness, soreness of the loin and knees, dim complexion due to deficiency of kidney yin and liver blood.

**Recipe 5**

**Ingredients**

Radix Rehmanniae Praeparata, 60 g

Fructus Lycii, 60 g

Lignum Aquilariae Resinatum, 6 g

plain spirits, 1000 ml

**Process**  Cut the first three ingredients into pieces, soak them in plain spirits, seal the container and put it in a cool, dry place for ten days. Then filter the tincture with a piece of gauze, store it up for future administration.

**Directions**  Take 10 ml three times daily.

**Indications**  Early greying of hair, alopecia, amnesia, infertility due to deficiency of both liver and kidney yin.

**Recipe 6**

**Ingredients**

Radix Rehmanniae, 30 g

Radix Rehmanniae Praeparata, 30 g

Radix Asparagi, 30 g

Radix Ophiopogonis, 30 g

Poria, 30 g

Radix Ginseng, 30 g

plain spirits, 1000 ml

**Process** Pound the first six ingredients into pieces and soak them in plain spirits in an earthen jar, seal the jar and put it in a cool, dry place for three days. Then open the lid slightly, cook it over a slow fire until it boils, after it cools, filter the decoction and store it up for future administration.

**Directions** Take 10 ml before meals three times daily.

**Indication** Early greying of hair due to deficiency of both yin and yang.

**Recipe 7**
**Ingredients**
Arillus Longan, 250 g
Radix Polygoni Multiflori, 250 g
Caulis Spatholobi, 250 g
rice wine, 1500 ml

**Process** Soak the first three ingredients in rice wine, seal the container and put it in a cool, dry place for ten days. Shake the container once daily during soaking. Then filter the tincture and store it up for future administration.

**Directions** Take 15 ml twice daily.

**Indication** Early greying of hair.

## Section 7 Impetigo

Impetigo is one of the commonly encountered suppurative dermatoses. It is caused by the infection of staphylococci and streptococci. At the initial stage, herpes appear in the affected region. After their diabrosis, yellow pussy water flows out, and the region becomes an erosive surface, itching and aching. It is mostly caused by stagnation of noxious dampness with invasion of pathogenic wind.

**Recipe**
**Ingredients**
Pericarpium Zanthoxyli, 10 g
vinegar, a right amount
plain spirits, a right amount

**Process** Grind bunge pricklyash peel into powder and mix it with a right amount of vinegar and plain spirits.

**Directions** Apply the mixture on the affected areas, three to five times daily. One course consisting of three days.

**Indication** Itching due to impetigo.

## Section 8 Scleroderma

Scleroderma is embraced in sclerosis, when fibrosis affects the skin, scleroderma occurs. Tight, firm skin may be present several years before visceral involvement becomes apparent. Although the disease is not always progressive, the survival of these patients is determined by the severity of visceral involvement. This disease is refractory and the subsequent prescription can only take some temporary and local effects by improving the patient's constitution, immunity, etc..

**Recipe 1**
**Ingredients**
Ganoderma Lucidum, 50 g
rice wine, 2500 ml
**Process**  Soak the first ingredient in rice wine and seal the container, put it in a cool, dry place for one week.
**Directions**  Take 10 ml twice daily.
**Indication**  Scleroderma.

**Recipe 2**
**Ingredients**
Radix Aconiti Praeparata, 60 g
mutton, 1000 g
Rhizoma Zingiberis, 100 g
Pericarpium Zanthoxyli, a right amount
Cortex Cinnamomi, 20 g
millet wine, a right amount
**Process**  Decoct aconite root for more than one hour first. Cook the above ingredients in a right amount of water over a slow fire until the meat is done.
**Directions**  Take the meat within one day. Contraindicated for cases with tachycardia.
**Indication**  Scleroderma.

**Recipe 3**
**Ingredients**
Monopterus Albus, 1
Radix Astragali, 15 g
Radix Angelicae Sinensis, 15 g
millet wine, a right amount
**Process**  Cut the finless eel open and remove the internal organs, wash it clean and cook it with

the other ingredients in a right amount of water.

**Directions**    Take the eel and the soup once daily.
**Indication**    Scleroderma.

**Recipe** 4
**Ingredients**
Radix Codonopsis Pilosulae, 30 g
Radix Astragali, 30 g
Cornu Cervi, 60 g
Herba Cistanchis, 30 g
millet wine, 1000 ml

**Process**    Soak the first four ingredients in millet wine, seal the container and put it in a cool, dry place for ten days. Then filter the tincture and store the extracts up for future administration.

**Directions**    Take 10 ml at bedtime daily.
**Indication**    Scleroderma.

# Chapter Seven
# Medicated Liquor for Nourishments and Longevity

## Section 1 Hypomnesis

Hypomnesis considered here is one of the presentations of senilism. In traditional Chinese medicine, it is concerned with insufficiency of kidney essence in combination with deficiency of heart blood and spleen qi.

**Recipe 1**
**Ingredients**
Radix Polygalae, 36 g
Radix Rehmanniae Praeparata, 36 g
Semen Cuscutae, 36 g
Fructus Schisandrae Chinensis, 36 g
Rhizoma Acori Graminei, 24 g
Rhizoma Chuanxiong, 24 g
Cortex Lycii Radicis, 48 g
plain spirits, 1200 ml

**Process** Pound and grind the first seven ingredients into powder and fill a gauze bag with it. Soak the bag in plain spirits and seal the container. Place the container in a cool, dry place for 7 days. Shake it once daily during soaking. Then take the bag out and filter the tincture, store the extracts up for future administration.

**Directions** Take 10 ml twice daily.

**Indications** Hypomnesis, accompanied with insomnia, dreaminess, palpitation or severe palpitation, dizziness, tinnitus, soreness of the waist and knees due to deficiency of kidney yin.

**Recipe 2**
**Ingredients**
Rhizoma Acori Graminei, 250 g
Rhizoma Atractylodis Macrocephalae, 250 g
plain spirits, 1500 ml

**Process** Cut grassleaved sweetflag rhizomes into pieces and steam them until they are done. Cut bighead atractylodes rhizomes into narrow pieces and fill them along with grassleaved sweetflag rhizomes in a gauze bag. Soak the bag in plain spirits and seal the container. Place the container in a cool, dry place for 7 days (in summer) or 14 days (in winter). Then take the bag out and filter the tincture, store the extracts up for future administration.

**Directions**  Take 10 ml twice daily.

**Indications**  Hypomnesis accompanied with irritability, restlessness, night sweat, insomnia, hectic fever due to deficiency of kidney yin resulting in abnormal ascending of asthenic fire.

### Recipe 3
**Ingredients**
Radix Ginseng, 36 g
lard, 360 g
old spirits, 4000 ml

**Process**  Grind ginger into fine powder for later use. Put the lard in a pot and heat it over a slow fire until the lard dissolves. Put spirits and dissolved lard in an earthen jar, add the powder of ginger in and stir the mixture equally. Seal the jar and place it in a cool, dry place for 21 days.

**Directions**  Take 10 ml twice daily.

**Indications**  Hypomnesis, general weakness.

### Recipe 4
**Ingredients**
Radix Polygalae, 10 g
plain spirits, 500 ml

**Process**  Grind polygala root into fine powder and soak it in plain spirits. Seal the container and place it in a cool, dry place for 7 days. Shake the container once daily during soaking.

**Directions**  Take 10 ml twice daily.

**Indications**  Hypomnesis, insomnia, palpitation, furuncle, carbuncle.

### Recipe 5
**Ingredients**
Folium Pini, 150 g
Herba Lophatheri, 75 g
Mel, 90 g
plain spirits, 1500 ml

**Process**  Wash the first two ingredients clean and cut them into pieces, dry them in the sun. Soak them along with honey in plain spirits and stir the mixture well. Seal the container for 30 days. Then remove the dregs and store the extracts up for future use.

**Directions**  Take 10 ml twice daily.

**Indications**  Hypomnesis, arteriosclerosis.

## Recipe 6
**Ingredients**
Arillus Longan, 250 g
sweet-scented osmanthus, 60 g
white sugar, 120 g
plain spirits, 2500 g

**Process**  Soak the first three ingredients in plain spirits and seal the container for six months.

**Directions**  Take 20 ml twice daily.

**Indications**  Hypomnesis, insomnia, dreaminess, palpitation, listlessness.

## Recipe 7
**Ingredients**
Semen Coicis, 100 g
Semen Sesami Nigrum, 125 g
Radix Rehmanniae, 125 g
plain spirits, 3000 ml

**Process**  Cook black sesames until they are done, dry them in the sun for later use. Stir-fry coix seeds until they become yellowish. Cut rehmannia root into small cubes. Pound prepared black sesames and coix seeds into powder and fill it along with rehmannia root in a gauze bag, fasten the mouth of it. Soak the bag in plain spirits and seal the container, place it in a cool, dry place for 21 days.

**Directions**  Take 20 ml before meals, twice daily.

**Indications**  Hypomnesis, weak constitution, listlessness, lassitude and fatigue, lumbocrural pain, xerosis cutis.

## Recipe 8
**Ingredients**
Cortex Albiziae, 100 g
millet wine, 500 ml

**Process**  Cut albizia barks into pieces, soak them in millet wine, seal the container and place it in a cool, dry place for 14 days. Shake the container once daily during soaking. Then filter the tincture and store the extracts up for future administration.

**Directions**  Take 20 ml before meals, twice daily.

**Indications**  Hypomnesis, neurosis, insomnia, headache, traumata.

## Section 2 Senile Lassitude in the Loin and Legs

Senile lassitude is due to deficiency of the qi and blood along with insufficiency of the kidney essence. The following prescriptions are effective for improving the symptoms of soreness of the waist and knees, weakness of the feet, etc..

**Recipe 1**
**Ingredients**
Agkistrodon acutus, 1
plain spirits, 500 ml
**Process**    Soak the snake in plain spirits and seal the container for 7 days. Remove the snake and store the extracts for administration.
**Directions**    Take 10 ml twice daily.
**Indications**    Lassitude in the loins and legs, dyskinesia.

**Recipe 2**
**Ingredients**
Semen Gossypii, 500 g
Fructus Psoraleae, 250 g
Semen Cuscutae, 250 g
Mel, a right amount
millet wine, a right amount
**Process**    Soak cotton seeds in boiling water for 10 minutes. Then dry them in the sun. Remove the oil from the shelled cotton seeds and soak them in millet wine in a port for 12 hours. Then cover the lid and steam the pot in boiling water for three to four hours. Take the seeds out and dry them again in the sun. Grind them along with psoralea fruit and dodder seeds into fine powder. Mix it with a right amount of honey to make pills. Each pill weighs 6 grams.
**Directions**    Take one pill twice daily.
**Indications**    Senile lassitude of loins and legs, frequency of micturition.

**Recipe 3**
**Ingredients**
Fructus Foenicuii, 30 g
Macrobracium Nipponense, 120 g
millet wine, a right amount
**Process**    Stir-fry common fennel fruit and grind them into fine powder. Pound the shrimps into mash and mix it with the powder of common fennel fruit to make pills. Each pill weighs 3 grams.
**Directions**    Take one pill with warm millet wine, twice daily.

**Indications**   Senile lassitude of loins and legs.

### Recipe 4
**Ingredients**
Cortex Acanthopanacis Radicis, 100 g
plain spirits, 500 ml
**Process**   Soak acanthopanax barks in plain spirits for two weeks.
**Directions**   Take 20 ml of the tincture once other day.
**Indications**   Senile lassitude of loins and legs.

### Recipe 5
It is the same as **Recipe 7** in Hypomnesis.
**Indications**   Senile lassitude of loins and legs, contractive pain in the lower extremities.

### Recipe 6
**Ingredients**
Folium Artemisiae, 20 g
pig trotter, 1
millet wine, 1000 ml
**Process**   Cook the first two ingredients in millet wine until the trotter is done.
**Directions**   Take the trotter once other day.
**Indications**   Senile lassitude of loins and legs.

### Recipe 7
**Ingredients**
Rhizoma Dioscoreae, 250 g
Mel, 20 g
millet wine, 1500 ml
**Process**   Wash Chinese yams clean and soak them in 500 ml of millet wine in a pot. Cook Chinese yams over a slow fire. Add in the surplus millet wine during the course of cooking until the yams are done. Take the yams out and pound them into mash, mix it with honey equally.
**Directions**   Take 50 g of the mixture twice daily.
**Indications**   Senile lassitude of loins and legs.

### Recipe 8
**Ingredients**
Pseudosciaena Polyactis, 30 g
Cornu Cervi, 30 g
millet wine, a right amount
**Process**   Stir-fry the first two ingredients until they become brown. Grind them into powder

and store up for future administration.

    **Directions**    Take 3 g with warm millet wine twice daily.

    **Indications**    Senile lassitude of loins and legs, lumbago due to deficiency of kidney yang.

**Recipe 9**
**Ingredients**
Rhizoma Cibotii, 20 g
Medulla Tetrapanacis, 12 g
Herba Verbenae, 12 g
Cortex Eucommiae, 15 g
Radix Dipsaci, 15 g
Radix Clematidis, 10 g
Radix Cyathulae, 6 g
plain spirits, 1000 ml

**Process**    Soak the first seven ingredients in plain spirits and seal the container for seven days.

**Directions**    Take 20 ml of the tincture once daily.

**Indications**    Lassitude of the loins and legs.

**Recipe 10**
**Ingredients**
Radix Morindae Officinalis, 30 g
Radix Achyranthis Bidentatae, 30 g
millet wine, 500 ml

**Process**    Soak the first two ingredients in millet wine and seal the container for seven days.

**Directions**    Take 10 ml of the tincture once daily.

**Indications**    Lassitude of the lower extremities.

**Recipe 11**
**Ingredients**
Excrementa Bombycum, 60 g
rice wine, 500 ml

**Process**    Soak silkworm excrement in rice wine in a pot. Cover the lid and cook it over a slow until it boils. Filter the decoction and store the extracts up for future administration.

    **Directions**    Take 25 ml once daily.

    **Indications**    Lassitude of the extremities, dyskinesia.

# Section 3  Deficiency of Yang

Deficiency of yang refers to yang shortage of spleen, heart and kidney. Deficiency of kidney yang is mainly considered in this chapter, which is manifested by giddiness, lassitude or cold pain in the loins and knees, impotence, premature ejaculation, sterility in women, clear urine, loose stool, pale complexion, listlessness, pale tongue, deep thready and feeble pulse.

**Recipe** 1
**Ingredients**
Radix Ginseng Rubra, 20 g
Cornu Cervi Pantotrichum, 6 g
plain spirits, 1000 ml

**Process**  Steam the first two ingredients until they become soft. After they cools, soak them in plain spirits, seal the container and put the container in a cool, dry place for 15 days.

**Directions**  Take 10 ml of the tincture twice daily.

**Indications**  Deficiency of yang manifested by aversion to cold, cold limbs. Contraindicated in summers.

**Recipe** 2
**Ingredients**
Radix Astragali, 60 g
Fructus Schisandrae Chinensis, 60 g
Rhizoma Dioscoreae Hypoglaucae, 45 g
Radix Ledebouriellae, 45 g
Rhizoma Chuanxiong, 45 g
Radix Achyranthis Bidentatae, 45 g
Radix Angelicae Pubescentis, 30 g
Fructus Corni, 30 g
plain spirits, 1500 ml

**Process**  Grind the first eight ingredients into powder and fill it in a gauze bag, fasten its mouth and soak in plain spirits, seal the container and put in a cool, dry place for three (in spring and summer) or five days (in autumn and winter). Remove the dregs and store the tincture up for future administration.

**Directions**  Take 10 ml before meals twice daily.

**Indications**  Deficiency of yang manifested by cold limbs, cold pain in the waist and knees.

**Recipe** 3
**Ingredients**

Herba Epimedii, 60 g

Fructus Psoraleae, 30 g

Radix Angelicae Sinensis, 30 g

Semen Cuscutae, 30 g

Fructus Rosae Laevigatae, 150 g

Radix Angelicae Pubescentis, 15 g

Radix Chuanxiong, 15 g

Radix Morindae Officinalis, 15 g

Fructus Foenicuii, 15 g

Cortex Cinnamomi, 15

Cortex Eucommiae, 15

Lignum Aquilariae Resinatum, 8 g

plain spirits, 4500 m

**Process**　Stir-fry psoralea fruit and common fennel fruit until they become yellowish. Fill the first twelve ingredients in a gauze bag and fasten its mouth. Soak it in plain spirits in a pot, cover its lid and steam the pot in boiling water for three hours. After it cools, seal the pot and put it in a cool, dry place for three days.

**Directions**　Take 20 ml of the tincture twice daily.

**Indications**　Deficiency of yang manifested by cold limbs, listlessness, lassitude and fatigue, emission, impotency, premature ejaculation. Also suitable for cases with deficiency of both qi and blood.

**Recipe** 4
**Ingredients**
Cornu Cervi Pantotrichum, 10 g

Cordyceps, 45 g

plain spirits, 800 ml

**Process**　Cut the first two ingredients into thin slices. Soak them in plain spirits, seal the container and put it in a cool, dry place for ten days. Shake the container once daily during the course of soaking. Then filter the tincture and store up for future administration.

**Directions**　Take 20 ml once daily.

**Indications**　Deficiency of kidney yang and insufficiency of essence and blood manifested by cold limbs, listlessness, lassitude and fatigue, emission, impotency, premature ejaculation. Contraindicated for cases with deficiency of yin.

**Recipe** 5
**Ingredients**
Colla Cornu Cervi, 80 g

plain spirits, 800 ml

**Process**　Grind antler glue into fine powder and soak it in a right amount of plain spirits (just inundate the powder with plain spirits) in an earthenware pot. Cook it over a slow fire. Keep on adding plain spirits in the pot during cooking until the powder dissolves thoroughly and 500 ml of decoction retained. After it cools, store the decoction up in a clean bottle for future administration.

**Directions**  Take 15 ml at bedtime, daily.

**Indications**  Lassitude of the loins and legs due to insufficiency of essence and blood, emission, metrorrhagia, leukorrhagia due to deficiency of kidney qi.

## Recipe 6
**Ingredients**
Herba Cistanchis, 60 g
Semen Myristicae, 30 g
Fructus Corni, 30 g
Cinnabaris, 10 g
plain spirits, 1200 ml

**Process**  Grind cinnabar into fine powder for later use. Pound the first three ingredients into pieces and fill them in a gauze bag, soak it in plain spirits, add the powder of cinnabar in and stir equally, seal the container and put it in a cool, dry place for seven days. Shake the container several times daily during soaking. Then remove the bag and store the tincture up for future administration.

**Directions**  Take 10 ml before meals twice daily.

**Indications**  Lassitude, soreness of the waist, emission, anorexia, epigastric pain, diarrhea due to deficiency of both spleen yang and kidney yang.

## Recipe 7
**Ingredients**
Gecko, 2
Radix Morindae Officinalis, 20 g
Ootheca Mantidis, 20 g
Radix Ginseng, 30 g
Herba Cistanchis, 30 g
Cornu Cervi Pantotrichum, 6 g
plain spirits, 2000 ml

**Process**  Cut pilose antler into thin slices; cut ginseng into thin pieces; remove the heads and feet of the geckoes and cut into small cubes; grind morinda root, desertliving cistanche herbs and mantis egg-cases into powder. Fill a gauze bag with the first six ingredients and fasten its mouth. Soak the bag in plain spirits and seal the container, put it in a cool, dry place for fourteen days. Shake the container several times daily during soaking. Then remove the bag and store the tincture up for future administration.

**Directions**  Take 10 ml before meals twice daily.

**Indications**  Lassitude of the lower extremities, listlessness, shortness of breath, dyspnea, insomnia, amnesia, palpitation, emission, cold pain in the loins and knees, infertility in women due to impairment of primordial vital energy and deficiency of kidney yang.

**Recipe** 8
**Ingredients**
Radix Angelicae Sinensis, 9 g
Fructus Lycii, 9 g
Fructus Psoraleae, 9 g
plain spirits, 1000 ml

**Process**   Pound the first ingredients into pieces and fill them in a gauze bag, soak it in plain spirits in a pot, cover its lid and steam the pot in boiling water for half one hour. After it cools, seal the pot and place it in a cool, dry place for 24 hours. Remove the bag and store the tincture up for future administration.

**Directions**   Take 10 to 20 ml twice daily.

**Indications**   Lassitude, lumbago, emission, dizziness due to deficiency of kidney yang and insufficiency of essence and blood.

## Section 4 Deficiency of qi

Deficiency of qi (vital energy) refers in traditional Chinese medicine mainly to the deficiency of lung and spleen. The organ lung controls the circulation of qi and spleen produces it. Hence hypofunction of the two organs can lead to general deficiency of qi. The condition is manifested by listlessness, spontaneous perspiration, dyspnea due to activities, anorexia, loose stools, diarrhea, pallor, pale tongue with white coating, slow and weak pulse.

**Recipe** 1
**Ingredients**
Radix Ginseng Alba, 30 g
plain spirits, 500 ml

**Process**   Cut white ginseng into thin slices and soak them in plain spirits, seal the container and put it in a cool, dry place for seven days. Shake the container once daily during soaking.

**Directions**   Take 10 ml twice daily. Add in the same amount of plain spirits as that of the tincture taken out from the container in the mean time.

**Indications**   Anorexia, dyspnea due to mild activities, lassitude and fatigue, spontaneous perspiration, insomnia, dreaminess, palpitation, amnesia, neurosis, pallor due to deficiency of lung qi and spleen qi.

### Recipe 2
**Ingredients**

Rhizoma Atractylodis Macrocephalae, 50 g

Radix Ginseng, 40 g

Rhizoma Dioscoreae, 40 g

Fructus Corni, 30 g

Fructus Schisandrae Chinensis, 30 g

Fructus Crataegi, 30 g

Rhizoma Zingiberis, 20 g

plain spirits, 2500 ml

**Process** Pound the first seven ingredients into pieces and fill them in a gauze bag, fasten its mouth, soak it in plain spirits and seal the container, put it in a cool, dry place for three weeks. Shake the container several daily during soaking.

**Directions** Take 10 ml three times daily.

**Indications** Anorexia, cold limbs, diarrhea, emission, dyspnea due to deficiency of spleen qi and kidney qi.

### Recipe 3
**Ingredients**

Radix Ginseng, 30 g

Radix Rehmanniae, 30 g

Poria, 30 g

Rhizoma Atractylodis Macrocephalae, 30 g

Radix Paeoniae Alba, 30 g

Radix Angelicae Sinensis, 30 g

Semen Oryzae cum Monasco, 30 g

Rhizoma Chuanxiong, 15 g

Arillus Longan, 120 g

crystal sugar, 250 g

plain spirits, 2000 ml

**Process** Pound the first nine ingredients into pieces and fill them in a gauze bag, fasten its mouth, soak it in plain spirits and seal the container, put it in a cool, dry place for four days. Shake the container several daily during soaking. Then remove the bag and add in crystal sugar for use.

**Directions** Take 10 to 15 ml three times daily.

**Indications** Lassitude and fatigue, anorexia, emaciation with sallow complexion, palpitation, shortness of breath due to deficiency of spleen qi and insufficiency of qi and blood.

### Recipe 4
**Ingredients**

Radix Ginseng Alba, 20 g

Rhizoma Atractylodis Macrocephalae, 20 g

Rhizoma Dioscoreae, 20 g

plain spirits, 500 ml

**Process**  Pound the first three ingredients into pieces and fill them in a gauze bag, fasten its mouth, soak it in plain spirits in an earthenware pot, cover the lid and cook it over a slow fire until it has been brought to hundreds of times of boils. After it cools, seal the container and put in a cool, dry place for 3 days. Remove the bag and filter the tincture, store it up for future administration.

**Directions**  Take 10 ml before meals three times daily.

**Indications**  Emaciation with sallow complexion, lassitude and fatigue, anorexia due to deficiency of spleen qi.

## Recipe 5
**Ingredients**

Radix Astragali, 120 g

rice wine, 1000 ml

**Process**  Pound milkvetch root into pieces and fill them in a gauze bag, fasten its mouth, soak it in rice wine, seal the container and put in a cool, dry place for 7 days. Shake the container once or twice daily during soaking. Remove the bag and filter the tincture, store it up for future administration.

**Directions**  Take 15 ml twice daily.

**Indications**  Anorexia, indigestion, palpitation, shortness of breath, lassitude of the extremities, profuse perspiration, prolapse of rectum due to deficiency of spleen qi and stomach qi.

## Recipe 6
**Ingredients**

Radix Codonopsis Pilosulae, 25 g

Fructus Lycii, 25 g

rice wine, 500 ml

**Process**  Cut pilose Asiabell root into slices and dry wolfberries in the sun. Soak them in rice wine, seal the container and put in a cool, dry place for 7 days. Remove the bag and filter the tincture, store it up for future administration.

**Directions**  Take 15 ml twice daily.

**Indications**  Anorexia, distention of the epigastric region after meals, lassitude of the extremities, soreness of the waist, dizziness, sallow complexion due to deficiency of spleen qi and stomach qi in combination with deficiency of blood.

## Recipe 7
**Ingredients**

Radix Codonopsis Pilosulae, 22.5 g

Radix Rehmanniae, 22.5

Poria, 22.5 g

Rhizoma Atractylodis Macrocephalae, 15 g

Radix Paeoniae Alba, 15 g

Semen Oryzae cum Monasco, 15 g

Radix Angelicae Sinensis, 15 g

Rhizoma Chuanxiong, 7.5 g

sweet-scented osmanthus, 125 g

Arillus Longan, 60 g

crystal sugar, 375

plain spirits, 4000 ml

**Process**   Grind the first ten ingredients into powder and fill it in a gauze bag, fasten its mouth, soak it in plain spirits, seal the container and put it in a cool, dry place for five days. Remove the bag and filter the tincture, add crystal sugar in and stir equally, store it up for future administration.

**Directions**   Take 10 ml twice daily.

**Indications**   Lassitude, shortness of breath, anorexia, insomnia and dreaminess, dyskinesia, pallor due to deficiency of spleen qi and heart qi in combination with insufficiency of both qi and blood.

### Recipe 8
**Ingredients**

Radix Codonopsis Pilosulae, 35 g

Radix Astragali, 35 g

plain spirits, 600 ml

**Process**   Soak the first two ingredients in plain spirits and seal the container, put it in a cool, dry place for 15 days.

**Directions**   Take 15 ml twice daily.

**Indications**   Lassitude, shortness of breath, dyspnea, spontaneous perspiration, aversion to wind due to deficiency of lung qi and spleen qi.

### Recipe 9
**Ingredients**

Rhizoma Atractylodis Macrocephalae, 200 g

plain spirits, 700 ml

**Process**   Pound bighead atractylodes rhizomes into pieces, put them in an earthenware pot, add in 600 ml of water, decoct them until 300 ml of decoction retained. Put the decoction and dregs in another container and add in plain spirits. Seal the container and put it in a cool, dry place for seven days. Filter the tincture with a piece of gauze and store the extracts up for future administration.

**Directions**   Take 10 ml twice daily.

**Indications**   Anorexia, distention and fullness sensation in the chest and abdomen, diarrhea due to deficiency of spleen qi and stomach qi.

**Recipe 10**
**Ingredients**
Rhizoma Polygonati, 40 g
plain spirits, 1000 ml

**Process**　　Wash Siberian solomonseal rhizomes clean and cut them into pieces, dry them in the sun and fill in a gauze bag, fasten the mouth and soak it in plain spirits, seal the container and put it in a cool, dry place for one month. Filter the tincture with a piece of gauze and store the extracts up for future administration.

**Directions**　　Take 15 ml twice daily.

**Indications**　　Lassitude and fatigue, arthralgia due to deficiency of qi and blood.

**Recipe 11**
**Ingredients**
Poria, 50 g
Flos Chrysanthemi, 50 g
Rhizoma Acori Graminei, 50 g
Radix Asparagi, 50 g
Rhizoma Atractylodis Macrocephalae, 50 g
Rhizoma Polygonati, 50 g
Radix Rehmanniae, 50 g
Radix Ginseng, 30 g
Cortex Cinnamomi, 30 g
Radix Achyranthis Bidentatae, 30 g
plain spirits, 2000 ml

**Process**　　Pound the first ten ingredients into powder and fill it in a gauze bag, fasten its mouth, soak it in plain spirits, seal the container and put it in a cool, dry place for 3 (in spring and summer) or 5 days (in autumn and winter). Filter the tincture with a piece of gauze and store the extracts up for future administration.

**Directions**　　Take 5 ml before meals twice daily.

**Indications**　　Lassitude and fatigue, general weakness, sallow complexion due to deficiency of qi.

**Recipe 12**
**Ingredients**
Radix Astragali, 75 g
Radix Codonopsis Pilosulae, 75 g
Rhizoma Polygonati Odorati, 75 g
Fructus Lycii, 75 g
Flos Carthami, 45 g

plain spirits, 5000 ml

**Process**   Cut the first five ingredients into pieces and fill them in a gauze bag, fasten its mouth, soak it in plain spirits, seal the container and put it in a cool, dry place for one month. Filter the tincture with a piece of gauze and store the extracts up for future administration.

**Directions**   Take 30 ml twice daily.

**Indications**   Lassitude and fatigue, listlessness due to deficiency of spleen qi and incoordination between qi and blood.

**Recipe** 13

**Ingredients**

Radix Astragali, 40 g

Rhizoma Polygonati, 40 g

Rhizoma Polygonati Odorati, 40 g

Cortex Eucommiae, 40 g

Fructus Lycii, 40 g

Radix Rehmanniae Praeparata, 40 g

Rhizoma Chuanxiong, 15 g

Radix Angelicae Sinensis, 20 g

Fructus Jujubae, 50 g

Radix Polygoni Multiflori, 25 g

Semen Cuscutae, 25 g

plain spirits, 2500 ml

**Process**   Grind the first eleven ingredients into powder and fill it in a gauze bag, fasten its mouth, soak it in plain spirits, seal the container and put it in a cool, dry place for two weeks. Filter the tincture with a piece of gauze and store the extracts up for future administration.

**Directions**   Take 30 ml twice daily.

**Indications**   Lassitude and fatigue, shortness of breath after mild activities, cold pain in the back, loins and knees due to deficiency of spleen qi and kidney qi.

## Section 5 Deficiency of Blood

Deficiency of blood considered here embraces deficiency of liver blood in combination with deficiency of spleen qi and heart blood which manifest a group of symptoms such as dizziness, palpitation, hypomenorrhea, delayed menstrual cycles, amenorrhea, pallor or sallow complexion, pale tongue, thready pulse etc.. The following prescriptions can be applied for cases with anemia, cancer, hematopathy which manifest the above syndromes.

### Recipe 1
**Ingredients**
Radix Rehmanniae, 60 g

plain spirits, 500 ml

**Process**  Wash rehmannia root clean and cut into thin slices, soak them in plain spirits and seal the container, put it in a cool, dry place for over seven days. Then remove the dregs and store the tincture for future administration.

**Directions**  Take 15 ml at bedtime, daily.

**Indications**  Numbness of the limbs, palpitation, consumption, hematemesis, epistaxis, metrorrhagia, traumata due to deficiency of blood. Contraindicated for cases with loose stools, cold limbs and distention of the abdomen.

### Recipe 2
**Ingredients**
Radix Rehmanniae, 1250 g

Semen Oryzae Glutinosae, 1250 g

distiller's yeast, 125 g

rice wine, 2500 ml

**Process**  Grind distiller's yeast into powder for later use. Pound rehmannia root into pieces, mix them with washed polished glutinous rice equally, put the mixture in an earthenware pot and stir-fry it until it is done. After the mixture cools, put it in an earthen jar, add in the powder of distiller's yeast and stir well, add rice wine in and seal the jar. Put it in a cool, dry place for ten days. Then remove the dregs and filter with a gauze bag, store the extracts for future administration.

**Directions**  Take 10 ml twice daily.

**Indications**  Lassitude and fatigue, dizziness, tinnitus, indigestion, irregular menstruation, early greying of hair due to deficiency of both yin and blood.

### Recipe 3
**Ingredients**
Radix Rehmanniae Praeparata, 120 g

Fructus Lycii, 60 g

Lignum Santali, 2 g

plain spirits, 1500 ml

**Process**  Pound the first three ingredients into pieces, fill them in a gauze bag, fasten its mouth, soak it in plain spirits and seal the container, put it in a cool, dry place for fourteen days.

**Directions**  Take 15 ml twice daily. Add in the same amount of plain spirits as that of the tincture taken for administration in the mean time.

**Indications**  Lassitude and fatigue, listlessness, impotency, soreness of the loins and knees, early greying of hair due to deficiency of both yin and blood.

### Recipe 4
**Ingredients**
Arillus Longan, 250 g
Radix Polygoni Multiflori, 250 g
Caulis Spatholobi, 250 g
rice wine, 1500 ml

**Process**   Cut suberect spatholobus stems and fleeceflower root into thin slices, pound longan fruit into pieces. Soak the first three ingredients in rice wine, seal the container, put it in a cool, dry place for ten days. Shake the container once to twice daily during soaking. Then remove the dregs and filter with a gauze bag, store the extracts for future administration.

**Directions**   Take 10 to 20 ml twice daily.

**Indications**   Lassitude of the extremities, dizziness, palpitation, insomnia, early greying of hair, pallor due to deficiency of both qi and blood. Contraindicated for cases with blood-heat or sthenic heat evil.

### Recipe 5
**Ingredients**
egg, 4
Colla Corii Asini, 40 g
salt, 10 g
rice wine, 500 ml

**Process**   Put rice wine in an earthen jar and cook it until it boils, add donkey-hide gelatin in. After it has dissolved, add yolks and salt in and stir equally, keep on cooking until it has been brought to several times of boils. Store the mixture up after it cools.

**Directions**   Take a right amount twice daily.

**Indications**   Lassitude and fatigue, cough due to consumption, hematemesis, hematochezia, threatened abortion, uterine hemorrhage during pregnancy, metrorrhagia, dysfunctional uterine bleeding, sallow complexion due to deficiency of blood.

### Recipe 6
**Ingredients**
Radix Polygoni Multiflori, 120 g
Radix Angelicae Sinensis, 60 g
Radix Rehmanniae, 80 g
Semen Sesami Nigrum, 60 g
plain spirits, 2500 ml

**Process**   Cut the first three ingredients into pieces and pound black sesame seeds into mash. Fill them in a gauze bag, fasten the mouth, put the bag in an earthen jar, add in plain spirits, cover the lid and cook it over a slow fire until it has been brought to several times of boils. After it cools, seal the jar and put it in a cool, dry place for seven days. Then remove the bag and filter the tincture with a piece of gauze, store the extracts up in a clean bottle for future administration.

**Directions**    Take 10 ml twice daily.

**Indications**    Aching pain in the loins and knees, emission, leukorrhagia, early greying of hair due to deficiency of both yin and blood resulted from insufficiency of liver and kidney.

**Recipe 7**
**Ingredients**
Fructus Lycii, 30 g
Arillus Longan, 30 g
Fructus Mori, 30 g
Fructus Jujubae, 50 g
plain spirits, 1000 ml

**Process**    Pound the first four ingredients into powder and soak them in plain spirits, seal the container and put it in a cool, dry place for fourteen days. Then remove the bag and filter the tincture with a piece of gauze, store the extracts up in a clean bottle for future administration.

**Directions**    Take 15 ml twice daily.

**Indications**    Dizziness, palpitation, lassitude and fatigue, shortness of breath, soreness of the loins and knees, anemia, neurosis due to deficiency of both yin and blood.

## Section 6  Deficiency of both Qi and Yin

Deficiency of both qi and yin refers to a syndrome comprising a group of presentations which occurs during the course of infectious diseases manifest mainly fever, come kind of chronic or consumptive diseases. These symptoms and signs are low-grade fever, feverish sensation in the palms and soles, spontaneous perspiration, night sweat, lassitude and fatigue, listlessness, dry mouth and throat, red tongue with little fur or without fur, weak, thready and rapid pulse etc.. The subsequent prescriptions have the efficacy of promoting qi and nourishing yin and can be applied for cases with the above syndrome.

**Recipe 1**
**Ingredients**
Radix Panacis Quinquefolii, 30 g
plain spirits, 500 ml

**Process**    Pound American ginseng into powder and soak it in plain spirits, seal the container and put it in a cool, dry place for fourteen days. Shake the container once daily during soaking.

**Directions**    Take 10 ml twice daily. Add in the same amount of plain spirits as that of the tincture administered in the mean time.

**Indications**   Lassitude and fatigue, hectic fever, chronic cough with no sputum, hemoptysis, dry mouth due to deficiency of both qi and yin. Contraindicated for cases with diarrhea of asthenic-cold type.

### Recipe 2
**Ingredients**

Radix Panacis Quinquefolii, 15 g

millet wine, 250 ml

plain spirits, 250 ml

**Process**   Wash American ginseng clean and dry it in the sun. Soak it in millet wine and plain spirits, seal the container and put it in a cool, dry place for ten days.

**Directions**   Take 25 ml twice daily.

**Indications**   Dry throat, chronic cough with no sputum, low-grade fever, fatigue due to deficiency of lung yin.

### Recipe 3
**Ingredients**

Radix Panacis Quinquefolii, 30 g

Radix Glehniae, 20 g

Radix Ophiopogonis, 20 g

millet wine, 800 ml

**Process**   Cut American ginseng and glehnia root into thin pieces and pound dwarf lilyturf tubers into pieces. Soak them in millet wine in an earthen jar, cover the lid, cook it over a slow fire until it boils. After the decoction cools, seal the jar and put it in a cool, dry place for seven days. Shake the jar once daily during soaking. Then add in 200 ml of cool boiled water and stir equally, filter the tincture with a pieces of gauze and store the extracts up for future administration.

**Directions**   Take 10 ml with warm boiled water, twice daily.

**Indications**   Irritability, thirst, chronic cough with no sputum due to deficiency of both qi and yin during the course of consumptive diseases.

### Recipe 4
**Ingredients**

Fructus Schisandrae Chinensis, 30 g

plain spirits, 500 ml

**Process**   Wash Chinese magnolcavine fruit clean and soak them in plain spirits, seal the container and put it in a cool, dry place for fourteen days.

**Directions**   Take 10 to 20 ml twice daily.

**Indications**   Chronic cough, thirst, spontaneous perspiration, chronic diarrhea, palpitation, insomnia, lassitude and fatigue due to deficiency of lung qi and yin.

**Recipe 5**
**Ingredients**
Radix Ginseng, 15 g
Fructus Lycii, 15 g
Rhizoma Dioscoreae, 15 g
Fructus Schisandrae Chinensis, 15 g
Radix Asparagi, 15 g
Radix Ophiopogonis, 15 g
Radix Rehmanniae, 15 g
Radix Rehmanniae Praeparata, 15 g
plain spirits, 3600 ml

**Process** Cut the first nine ingredients into thin slices and fill them in a gauze bag, fasten the mouth, soak it in plain spirits in an earthen jar, cover the lid and steam it in boiling water for half one hour. After it cools, seal the jar and put it in a cool, dry place for 10 days. Then filter the tincture and store the extracts up for future administration.

**Directions** Take 10 ml twice daily.

**Indications** Lassitude of the extremities, fatigue, soreness of the loins and legs, restlessness, thirst, palpitation, dreaminess, dizziness, early greying of hair due to deficiency of both qi and yin.

**Recipe 6**
**Ingredients**
Radix Asparagi, 500 g
Semen Oryzae Glutinosae, 750 g
distiller's yeast, 50 g

**Process** Grind distiller's yeast into powder for later use. Cook polished glutinous rice in water until it is half-done. Decoct lucid asparagus roots in a right amount of water until they are done. Put the decoction along with the dregs in an earthen jar, add the powder of distiller's yeast and polished glutinous rice in and stir equally. Seal the jar and put it in a dry place for seven days. Filter out the extracts with a pieces of gauze bag and store up for future administration.

**Directions** Take 10 ml three times daily.

**Indications** Cough, aching pain and numbness of the extremities due to deficiency of lung yin and kidney yin.

**Recipe 7**
**Ingredients**
Rhizoma Dioscoreae, 15 g
Fructus Corni, 15 g
Fructus Schisandrae Chinensis, 15 g
Ganoderma Lucidum, 15 g

plain spirits, 1000 ml

**Process**  Pound the first four ingredients into pieces and fill them in a gauze bag, fasten its mouth, soak it in plain spirits, seal the container and put it in a cool, dry place for one month. Shake the container several times daily during soaking. Then filter the tincture and store up for future administration.

**Directions**  Take 10 ml twice daily.

**Indications**  Cough, thirst, night sweat, emission due to deficiency of lung yin and kidney yin.

## Recipe 8
**Ingredients**

Herba Dendrobii Nobilis, 240 g

millet wine, 1000 ml

**Process**  Soak dendrobium stems in millet wine, seal the container and put it in a cool, dry place for seven days. Then filter the tincture and store up for future administration.

**Directions**  Take 15 ml twice daily.

**Indications**  Lassitude of the loins and legs, low-grade fever due to deficiency of both qi and yin

## Recipe 9
**Ingredients**

Semen Phaseoli Radiati, 30 g

Rhizoma Dioscoreae, 30 g

Cortex Phellodendri, 22 g

Radix Achyranthis Bidentatae, 22 g

Radix Scrophulariae, 22 g

Radix Glehniae, 22 g

Radix Paeoniae Alba, 22 g

Fructus Gardeniae, 22 g

Radix Asparagi, 22 g

Radix Ophiopogonis, 22 g

Radix Trichosanthis, 22 g

Radix Angelicae Sinensis, 18 g

Radix Glycyrrhizae, 4.5 g

plain spirits, 2500 ml

Mel, 30 g

**Process**  Pound the first thirteen ingredients into pieces and fill them in a gauze bag, fasten its mouth, soak it in plain spirits, seal the container and put it in a cool, dry place for fourteen days. Shake the container several times daily during soaking. Then filter the tincture and add in honey, stir the mixture well and store up for future administration.

**Directions**  Take 15 to 20 ml twice daily.

**Indications**  Cough with no sputum, dry mouth, irritability due to insufficiency of lung yin and fluid. Contraindicated for cases with hemoptysis and epistaxis.

## Section 7  Deficiency of both Qi and Blood

Deficiency of both qi and blood refers to a syndrome manifests a group of presentations such as listlessness, shortness of breath, anorexia, palpitation, dizziness, tinnitus, xerosis cutis, sallow complexion, etc.. The syndrome is due to long-term and recurrent diseases which consume qi and blood. The following prescriptions have the efficacy of both promoting qi and invigorating blood. They can be applied for cases with the above syndrome.

**Recipe** 1
**Ingredients**
Semen Biotae, 30 g
Radix Polygoni Multiflori, 30 g
Herba Cistanchis, 30 g
Radix Achyranthis Bidentatae, 30 g
plain spirits, 1000 ml

**Process**  Cut the first four ingredients into pieces and soak them in plain spirits, seal the container and put it in a cool, dry place for ten (in spring and summer) or twenty days. Shake the container several times daily during soaking. Then filter the tincture and store up for future administration.

**Directions**  Take 10 ml twice daily.
**Indications**  Palpitation, shortness of breath resulted from lack of qi and blood.

**Recipe** 2
**Ingredients**
Radix Ginseng, 5 g
Radix Rehmanniae Praeparata, 25 g
Fructus Lycii, 90 g
crystal sugar, 100 g
plain spirits, 2500 ml

**Process**  Cut ginger into thin slices, fill them along with rehmannia root and mulberries in a gauze bag, fasten its mouth, soak it in plain spirits, seal the container and put it in a cool, dry place for fifteen days. Shake the container once daily during soaking. Then filter the tincture out with a piece of gauze for later use. Put crystal sugar in a pot and add in a small amount of water, cook the sugar until it dissolves thoroughly, and add it in the filtered tincture, stir the mixture well and store up for future administration.

**Directions**  Take 15 ml twice daily.

**Indications**  Lassitude and fatigue, consumption, insomnia, dreaminess, anorexia due to lack of qi and blood especially that of the heart.

**Recipe** 3
**Ingredients**
Radix Angelicae Sinensis, 26 g
Rhizoma Atractylodis Macrocephalae, 26 g
Rhizoma Chuanxiong, 10 g
Radix Paeoniae Alba, 18 g
Radix Rehmanniae, 15 g
Radix Ginseng, 15 g
Poria, 20 g
Radix Glycyrrhizae, 20 g
Cortex Acanthopanacis Radicis, 25 g
Fructus Jujubae, 36 g
Semen Juglandis, 36 g
plain spirits, 1500 ml

**Process**  Grind the first eleven ingredients into fine powder and fill it in a gauze bag, soak it in plain spirits in an earthen jar, cover the lid and cook it over a slow fire for one hour. After it cools, seal the jar and put it in a cool, dry place for ten days. Remove the dregs and store the tincture up for future administration.

**Directions**  Take 10 ml before meals three times daily.

**Indications**  Lassitude and fatigue, listlessness, anorexia, emaciation with sallow complexion due to deficiency of qi and blood.

**Recipe** 4
**Ingredients**
Radix Angelicae Sinensis, 22 g
Rhizoma Chuanxiong, 7.5 g
Radix Paeoniae Alba, 15 g
Radix Glycyrrhizae Praeparata, 12 g
Cortex Acanthopanacis Radicis, 60 g
Fructus Jujubae, 30 g
Semen Juglandis, 30 g
rice wine, 5000 ml

**Process**  Cut the first seven ingredients into thin slices and fill them in a gauze bag, fasten its mouth, soak it in rice wine in an earthen jar, cover the lid and cook it over a slow fire for one hour. After it cools, seal the jar and put it in a cool, dry place for ten days. Remove the dregs and store the extracts up for future administration.

**Directions**  Take 15 to 20 ml three times daily.

**Indications**  Lassitude and fatigue, anorexia, dizziness, shortness of breath, hypomenorrhea accompanied with soreness of the loin and knees due to deficiency of qi and blood.

**Recipe** 5
**Ingredients**
Radix Asparagi, 30 g
Radix Ophiopogonis, 30 g
Radix Rehmanniae, 62 g
Radix Rehmanniae Praeparata, 62 g
Radix Ginseng, 15 g
Fructus Lycii, 15 g
Fructus Amomi, 5 g
Radix Aucklandiae, 3.8 g
Lignum Aquilariae Resinatum, 2.3 g
plain spirits, 4000 ml

**Process**  Grind the first nine ingredients into powder and fill it in a gauze bag, fasten its mouth, soak it in plain spirits in an earthen jar for three days, then steam it in boiling water over a slow fire for half one hour. After it cools, seal the jar and put it in a cool, dry place for two days. Remove the dregs and store the extracts up for future administration.

**Directions**  Take a right amount daily.

**Indications**  Lassitude and fatigue, listlessness, shortness of breath, anorexia, distention and fullness of the epigastric region, early greying of hair due to insufficiency of qi and blood in combination with disharmony between spleen and stomach.

**Recipe** 6
**Ingredients**
Fructus Lycii, 12 g
Radix Angelicae Sinensis, 15 g
Rhizoma Chuanxiong, 15 g
Radix Paeoniae Alba, 15 g
Radix Rehmanniae Praeparata, 15 g
Radix Ginseng, 15 g
Rhizoma Atractylodis Macrocephalae, 15 g
Poria, 15 g
Radix Glycyrrhizae, 15 g
Fructus Jujubae, 10 g
Rhizoma Zingiberis, 30 g
plain spirits, 6000 ml

**Process**   Pound the first eleven ingredients into pieces and fill them in a gauze bag, fasten its mouth, soak it in plain spirits in an earthen jar for 14 days. Then remove the dregs and store the extracts up for future administration.

**Directions**   Take 10 ml twice daily.

**Indications**   Lassitude and fatigue, early greying of hair, xerosis cutis, emaciation with sallow complexion due to insufficiency of qi and blood.

### Recipe 7
**Ingredients**
Radix Angelicae Sinensis, 25 g
Rhizoma Atractylodis Macrocephalae, 25 g
Cortex Acanthopanacis Radicis, 60 g
Radix Paeoniae Alba, 20 g
Poria, 15 g
Radix Glycyrrhizae, 12 g
Radix Ginseng, 10 g
Rhizoma Chuanxiong, 10 g
Semen Juglandis, 30 g
Fructus Jujubae, 30 g
Radix Rehmanniae, 30 g
rice wine, 5000 ml

**Process**   Cut the first eleven ingredients into pieces and fill them in a gauze bag, fasten its mouth, soak it in rice wine in an earthen jar, cover the lid and cook it over a slow fire for one hour and a half. After it cools, seal the jar and put it in a cool, dry place for twelve days. Remove the dregs and store the extracts up for future administration.

**Directions**   Take 10 ml warmly, three times daily.

**Indications**   Lassitude and fatigue, anorexia, loose stool, listlessness, irregular menstruation, metrorrhagia, emaciation with sallow complexion due to deficiency of qi and blood.

### Recipe 8
**Ingredients**
Fructus Psoraleae, 30 g
Radix Rehmanniae, 30 g
Radix Rehmanniae Praeparata, 30 g
Radix Asparagi, 30 g
Radix Ophiopogonis, 30 g
Radix Ginseng, 30 g
Radix Angelicae Sinensis, 30 g
Rhizoma Chuanxiong, 30 g
Radix Paeoniae Alba, 30 g

Poria, 30 g

Semen Biotae, 30 g

Fructus Amomi, 30 g

Rhizoma Acori Graminei, 30 g

Radix Polygalae, 30 g

Radix Aucklandiae, 15 g

plain spirits, 2000 ml

**Process**  Pound the first fifteen ingredients into pieces and fill them in a gauze bag, fasten its mouth, soak it in plain spirits in an earthen jar, cover the lid and cook it over a slow fire until it boils. After it cools, remove the dregs and store the extracts up for future administration.

**Directions**  Take 10 ml warmly, twice daily.

**Indications**  Severe palpitation, dizziness, amnesia due to deficiency of qi and blood.

**Recipe** 9

**Ingredients**

Radix Ginseng, 6 g

Radix Notoginseng, 18 g

Rhizoma Chuanxiong, 18 g

Radix Angelicae Sinensis, 60 g

Radix Astragali, 60 g

Cortex Acanthopanacis Radicis, 36 g

Rhizoma Atractylodis Macrocephalae, 36 g

Radix Glycyrrhizae, 12 g

Fructus Schisandrae Chinensis, 24 g

Poria, 24 g

plain spirits, 3000 m

**Process**  Cut the first ten ingredients into pieces and soak them in plain spirits and seal the container for over fifteen days.

**Directions**  Take 15 to 30 ml twice daily.

**Indications**  Fatigue and lassitude, general weakness, insomnia, dreaminess, anorexia due to deficiency of both qi and blood.

**Recipe** 10

**Ingredients**

Radix Ginseng, 40 g

Radix Angelicae Sinensis, 25 g

Semen Ziziphi Spinosae, 10 g

Radix Polygalae, 15 g

Arillus Longan, 20 g

Radix Rehmanniae, 20 g

crystal sugar, 40 g

plain spirits, 1500 ml

**Process**  Cut the first six ingredients into slices, fill them in a gauze bag, fasten its mouth, soak it in plain spirits, seal the container and put it in a cool, dry place for fourteen days. Shake the container once daily during soaking. Then filter the tincture out with a piece of gauze for later use. Put crystal sugar in a pot and add in a small amount of water, cook the sugar until it dissolves thoroughly, and add it in the filtered tincture, stir the mixture well and store up for future administration.

**Directions**  Take 10 ml twice daily.

**Indications**  Lassitude and fatigue, insomnia, amnesia, palpitation, dizziness, restlessness, anorexia, sallow complexion due to deficiency of both qi and blood especially that of the heart.

# Section 8
# Additional Prescriptions for Health Preserving

### Recipe 1
**Ingredients**

Radix Angelicae Sinensis, 30 g

Flos Chrysanthemi, 30 g

Arillus Longan, 240 g

Fructus Lycii, 120 g

plain spirits, 5000 ml

**Process**  Fill the first four ingredients in a gauze bag and fasten its mouth, soak it in plain spirits and seal the container, put it in a cool, dry place for over one month. Then remove the bag and store the tincture up for future administration.

**Directions**  Take 10 ml once or twice daily.

**Indications**  Dizziness, blurring of vision, insomnia, palpitation, amnesia, pallor due to insufficiency of blood and impairment of essence.

### Recipe 2
**Ingredients**

Radix Rehmanniae Praeparata, 120 g

Radix Angelicae Sinensis, 150 g

Rhizoma Chuanxiong, 45 g

Cortex Eucommiae, 45 g

Poria, 45 g

Radix Glycyrrhizae, 30 g

Fructus Rosae Laevigatae, 30 g

Herba Epimedii, 30 g

Herba Dendrobii, 90 g

plain spirits, 1500 ml

**Process**  Pound and grind the above ingredients into powder, fill them in a gauze bag and fasten its mouth, soak it in plain spirits and seal the container, put it in a cool, dry place for seven (in spring and summer) or fourteen days (in autumn and winter). Then remove the bag and store the tincture up for future administration.

**Directions**  Take 10 ml before meals, twice daily.

**Indications**  Consumption, anorexia emaciation with dusty complexion due to insufficiency of blood and essence, pallor, soreness of the loin and knees due to deficiency of kidney yang.

### Recipe 3
**Ingredients**
Rhizoma Polygonati, 150 g

Radix Polygoni Multiflori, 75 g

Fructus Lycii, 75 g

Semen Ziziphi Spinosae, 75 g

plain spirits, 1500 ml

**Process**  Cut Siberian solomonseal rhizomes and fleeceflower root into pieces, fill them along with wolfberries and spine date seed in a gauze bag and fasten its mouth, soak it in plain spirits and seal the container, put it in a cool, dry place for two months. Then remove the bag and store the tincture up for future administration.

**Directions**  Take 25 ml twice daily.

**Indications**  Dizziness, insomnia, lassitude and fatigue, anorexia due to deficiency of yin and blood especially that of the heart.

### Recipe 4
**Ingredients**
Fructus Lycii, 100 g

Arillus Longan, 100 g

Fructus Ligustri Lucidi, 100 g

Radix Rehmanniae, 100 g

Herba Epimedii, 100 g

Semen Phaseoli Radiati, 100 g

lard, 400 g

plain spirits, 5000 ml

**Process**  Cut the first six ingredients into pieces and fill them in a gauze bag and fasten its mouth, soak it in plain spirits and add dissolved lard in, stir the mixture equally, seal the container, put it in a cool, dry place for three weeks. Shake the container once other day during soaking. Then remove the bag and store the extracts up for future administration.

**Directions**   Take 10 ml before meals, three times daily.

**Indications**   Lassitude and fatigue, soreness of the waist, emission, dizziness, senile cough, arthralgia, dribbling urination (prostatic hyperplasia), distention and fullness sensation of the abdomen, xerosis cutis, palpitation due to deficiency of kidney qi in combination with deficiency of both heart qi and blood.

**Recipe** 5

**Ingredients**

Radix Rehmanniae, 15 g

Radix Rehmanniae Praeparata, 15 g

Radix Asparagi, 15 g

Radix Ophiopogonis, 15 g

Radix Angelicae Sinensis, 15 g

Radix Achyranthis Bidentatae, 15 g

Fructus Foenicuii, 15 g

Cortex Eucommiae, 15 g

Radix Morindae Officinalis, 15 g

Rhizoma Chuanxiong, 15 g

Radix Paeoniae Alba, 15 g

Fructus Lycii, 15 g

Herba Cistanchis, 15 g

Cortex Phellodendri, 15 g

Poria, 15 g

Rhizoma Anemarrhenae, 15 g

Fructus Psoraleae, 10 g

Fructus Amomi, 10 g

Rhizoma Atractylodis Macrocephalae, 10 g

Radix Polygalae, 10 g

Radix Ginseng, 10 g

Rhizoma Acori Graminei, 8 g

Semen Biotae, 8 g

Radix Aucklandiae, 6 g

plain spirits, 4500 ml

**Process**   Cut the above ingredients except plain spirits into pieces, fill them in a gauze bag and fasten its mouth, soak it in plain spirits in an earthen jar, cover the lid, cook it over a slow fire for two hours. After it cools, seal the jar and put it in a cool, dry place for twelve days. Then remove the bag and store the tincture up for future administration.

**Directions**   Take 15 ml twice daily.

**Indications**   Lassitude of the extremities, fatigue and listlessness, soreness of the loin and knees, emission, impotency, tinnitus, early greying of hair, emaciation with sallow complexion, insomnia, dreaminess, palpitation due to impairment of liver and kidney in combination with deficiency of qi and blood.

**Recipe** 6
**Ingredients**
Radix Rehmanniae, 30 g
Radix Rehmanniae Praeparata, 30 g
Radix Asparagi, 30 g
Radix Ophiopogonis, 30 g
Rhizoma Dioscoreae, 30 g
Semen Nelumbinis, 30 g
Fructus Jujubae, 30 g
plain spirits, 1500 ml

**Process**   Cut the first seven ingredients into small cubes and fill them in a gauze bag and fasten its mouth, soak it in plain spirits, seal the container and put it in a cool, dry place for fifteen days. Then remove the bag and store the tincture up for future administration.

**Directions**   Take 30 ml twice daily.

**Indications**   Listlessness, dizziness, blurring of vision, palpitation, amnesia, insomnia, dreaminess, anorexia, or hectic fever, constipation, polydipsia, early greying of hair due to insufficiency of liver yin and kidney yin and lack of heart blood along with deficiency of spleen qi and stomach qi.

**Recipe** 7
**Ingredients**
Semen Nelumbinis, 60 g
Semen Pini, 60 g
Semen Juglandis, 60 g
Semen Ginkgo, 60 g
Arillus Longan, 60 g
plain spirits, 3000 ml

**Process**   Pound the first five ingredients into pieces, fill them in a gauze bag and fasten its mouth, soak it in plain spirits, seal the container and put it in a cool, dry place for fifteen days. Then remove the bag and store the tincture up for future administration.

**Directions**   Take 10 ml twice daily.

**Indications**   Lassitude and fatigue due to mild activities, general weakness, palpitation, shortness of breath, anorexia due to deficiency of both yin and yang.

**Recipe** 8
**Ingredients**
Fructus Lycii, 120 g

Arillus Longan, 60 g

Radix Angelicae Sinensis, 30 g

Rhizoma Atractylodis Macrocephalae, 15 g

Semen Sojae Nigrum, 175 g

plain spirits, 3500 ml

**Process**   Pound black soya beans into pieces, fill the first five ingredients in a gauze bag and fasten its mouth, soak it in plain spirits, seal the container and put it in a cool, dry place for seven days. Then remove the bag and store the tincture up for future administration.

**Directions**   Take 20 ml twice daily.

**Indications**   General weakness, insomnia, dreaminess, xerosis cutis, emaciation with sallow complexion due to deficiency of yin and blood.

**Recipe** 9

**Ingredients**

Cortex Eucommiae, 50 g

Rhizoma Chuanxiong, 40 g

Radix Angelicae Sinensis, 100 g

Herba Dendrobii Nobilis, 100 g

Semen Cuscutae, 120 g

Radix Rehmanniae, 30 g

Rhizoma Alismatis, 30 g

Herba Epimedii, 30 g

plain spirits, 1500 ml

**Process**   Cut the first eight ingredients into pieces and fill them in a gauze bag and fasten its mouth, soak it in plain spirits, seal the container and put it in a cool, dry place for fourteen days. Shake the container several times daily during soaking. Then remove the bag and store the tincture up for future administration.

**Directions**   Take 15 to 20 ml twice daily.

**Indications**   Impotency, soreness and aching pain in the loin and knees, emaciation due to deficiency of liver yin and kidney essence or insufficiency of blood and essence.

**Recipe** 10

**Ingredients**

Radix Ginseng, 30 g

Fructus Litchi, 1000 g

plain spirits, 5000 ml

**Process**   Cut ginseng into thin slices and fill them along with litchi fruits in a gauze bag and fasten its mouth, soak it in plain spirits, seal the container and put it in a cool, dry place for three days. Shake the container several times daily during soaking.

**Directions**   Take 10 ml twice daily.

**Indications**   General weakness, listlessness.

**Recipe** 11
**Ingredients**
Radix Rehmanniae, 250 g
Fructus Lycii, 250 g
Flos Chrysanthemi, 250 g
Semen Oryzae Glutinosae, 2500 g
distiller's yeast, 200 g

**Process**   Cut the first three ingredients into pieces and grind distiller's yeast into fine powder. Put the pieces in an earthenware pot, add 5000 ml of water, cook the dregs over a slow fire until 2500 ml of decoction retained. Remove the dregs and store the decoction in an earthen jar for later use. Cook polished glutinous rice until it is done. Dry the rice in the sun. Mix the half-dried rice with the powder of distiller's yeast equally, then put the mixture in the jar, and mix it with the decoction equally. Seal the jar and put it in a thermal insulating place for three weeks. Filter the dregs and store the extracts for future administration.

**Directions**   Take 20 ml before meals three times daily.
**Indications**   Dizziness and early greying of hair due to insufficiency of liver and kidney.

**Recipe** 12
**Ingredients**
Radix Codonopsis Pilosulae, 20 g
Radix Rehmanniae Praeparata, 20 g
Fructus Lycii, 20 g
Semen Astragali Complanati, 15 g
Herba Epimedii, 15 g
Flos Caryophylli, 15 g
Radix Polygalae, 10 g
Fructus Litchi, 10 g
Lignum Aquilariae Resinatum, 6 g
plain spirits, 1000 ml

**Process**   Pound the first eight ingredients into pieces and eagle wood into powder. Fill them in a gauze bag and fasten its mouth, soak it in plain spirits, seal the container and put it in a cool, dry place for three days. Shake the container several times daily during soaking. Then open the lid of the container slightly and cook it over a slow fire until it has been brought to hundreds of times of boils. After it cools, seal the container and put it in a cool, dry place again for three weeks. After it is done, remove the bag and store the tincture up for future administration.

**Directions**   Take 10 ml before meals twice daily.
**Indications**   Lassitude and fatigue, impotency, emission, premature ejaculation, soreness of the loin and knees, dizziness, palpitation, shortness of breath, anorexia, hiccup, diarrhea, emaciation

with sallow complexion due to deficiency of kidney and insufficiency of blood along with deficiency of spleen qi and stomach qi.

**Recipe** 13
**Ingredients**
Fructus Jujubae, 300 g
Radix Angelicae Sinensis, 30 g
Rhizoma Acori Graminei, 15 g
Radix Curcumae, 15 g
Cortex Acanthopanacis Radicis, 15 g
Radix Achyranthis Bidentatae, 15 g
Pericarpium Citri Reticulatae, 15 g
Poria cum Ligno Hospite, 15 g
Radix Ophiopogonis, 15 g
Flos Carthami, 7.5 g
plain spirits, 3500 ml

**Process**  Cut the first ten ingredients into pieces and fill them in a gauze bag and fasten its mouth, soak it in plain spirits in an earthen jar, cover the lid and steam the jar in boiling water for two hours. After it cools, seal the jar and put it in a cool, dry place again for three weeks. Then remove the bag and store the tincture up for future administration.

**Directions**  Take 20 ml twice daily.

**Indications**  General weakness, lassitude and fatigue, emaciation, amnesia, insomnia, anorexia.

**Recipe** 14
**Ingredients**
Radix Achyranthis Bidentatae, 15 g
Fructus Lycii, 15 g
Radix Rehmanniae, 15 g
Cortex Eucommiae, 15 g
Flos Chrysanthemi, 15 g
Radix Paeoniae Alba, 15 g
Fructus Corni, 15 g
Fructus Chaeomelis, 7.5 g
Radix Angelicae Sinensis, 7.5 g
Cortex Acanthopanacis Radicis, 30 g
Ramulus Loranthi, 30 g
Ramulus Cinnamomi, 1.5 g
Arillus Longan, 60 g
plain spirits, 2000 ml

**Process** Cut the first thirteen ingredients into pieces and fill them in a gauze bag and fasten its mouth, soak it in plain spirits, seal the container and put it in a cool, dry place for one week. Then remove the bag and store the tincture up for future administration.

**Directions** Take 15 ml twice daily.

**Indications** Dizziness, lassitude and pain in the loin and knees, numbness of the extremities due to deficiency of liver blood and kidney essence.

**Recipe** 15
**Ingredients**
Fructus Lycii, 100 g
Succus Ophiopogonis, 60 g
Radix Rehmanniae, 100 g
Semen Armeniacae Amarum, 30 g
Radix Ginseng, 20 g
Poria, 30 g
plain spirits, 1500 ml

**Process** Pound ginseng, poria and bitter apricot seed into pieces and soak them along with the first three ingredients in plain spirits, seal the container and put it in a cool, dry place for one week. Then remove the dregs and store the tincture up for future administration.

**Directions** Take 10 ml warmly before meals, twice daily.

**Indication** Dim complexion.

**Recipe** 16
**Ingredients**
Radix Ginseng, 30 g
Radix Angelicae Sinensis, 30 g
Rhizoma Polygonati Odorati, 30 g
Rhizoma Polygonati, 30 g
Radix Polygoni Multiflori, 30 g
Fructus Lycii, 30 g
millet wine, 1500 ml

**Process** Cut the first five ingredients into pieces and soak them along with mulberries in millet wine, seal the container and put it in a cool, dry place for one week. Then remove the dregs and store the tincture up for future administration.

**Directions** Take 20 ml twice daily.

**Indications** Emaciation with sallow complexion, xerosis cutis.

**Recipe** 17
**Ingredients**
Flos Persicae, 250 g

Radix Angelicae Dahuricae, 30 g

plain spirits, 1000 ml

**Process**  Soak the first two ingredients in plain spirits, seal the container and put it in a cool, dry place for one month. Then remove the dregs and store the tincture up for future administration.

**Directions**  Spread 15 ml of the tincture over the affected parts of the face with rubbing method, twice daily.

**Indications**  Dusty complexion, chloasma. Contraindicated for cases during pregnancies.

**Recipe** 18

**Ingredients**

Semen Arecae, 20 g

Pericarpium Citri Reticulatae, 20 g

Pericarpium Citri Reticulatae Viride, 10 g

Flos Rosae Rugosae, 10 g

Fructus Amomi, 5 g

crystal sugar, 10 g

millet wine, 1500 ml

**Process**  Pound and grind the first five ingredients into powder and fill it in a gauze bag, fasten its mouth, soak it in millet wine in an earthen jar, cover the lid and cook it over a slow fire for thirty minutes. After it cools, remove the bag from the tincture. Add crystal sugar in the tincture and store the extracts up for future administration.

**Directions**  Take 20 ml twice daily.

**Indications**  Chloasma accompanied with anorexia, chest distress, hypochondriac pain, depressive emotion, irregular menstruation due to stagnation of liver qi.

**Recipe** 19

**Ingredients**

Radix Angelicae Sinensis, 15 g

Arillus Longan, 15 g

plain spirits, 500 ml

**Process**  Soak the first two ingredients in plain spirits, seal the container and put it in a cool, dry place for one week. Then remove the dregs and store the tincture up for future administration.

**Directions**  Take 15 ml at bedtime daily.

**Indications**  Xerosis cutis, senile plaques.

**Recipe** 20

**Ingredients**

Flos Chrysanthemi, 30 g

Radix Rehmanniae, 10 g

Radix Angelicae Sinensis, 10 g

Fructus Lycii, 20 g

plain spirits, 500 ml

**Process**   Wash the first three ingredients clean, fill them in a gauze bag, fasten its mouth, soak it in plain spirits, seal the container and put it in a cool, dry place for one week. Then remove the bag and store the tincture up for future administration.

**Directions**   Take 10 to 20 ml twice daily.

**Indications**   Dizziness, fatigue.

### Recipe 21
**Ingredients**

Arillus Longan, 30 g

crystal sugar, 100 g

plain spirits, 500 ml

**Process**   Soak the first two ingredients in plain spirits, seal the container and put it in a cool, dry place for one to three months. Then remove the dregs and store the tincture up for future administration.

**Directions**   Take 20 ml twice daily.

**Indication**   Applied for relieving fatigue.

### Recipe 22
**Ingredients**

Peni et Testes Callorhini, one set

Radix Ginseng, 15 g

Rhizoma Dioscoreae, 30 g

plain spirits, 1000 ml

**Process**   Cut ursine seal's penis and testes into slices and soak them along with ginseng and Chinese yams in plain spirits, seal the container and put it in a cool, dry place for seven days. Then remove the dregs and store the tincture up for future administration.

**Directions**   Take 10 ml twice daily.

**Indication**   Fatigue. Contraindicated for cases with conjunctival congestion, sore throat, cough with no sputum, hemoptysis, constipation due to deficiency of yin resulting in abnormal ascending of asthenic fire.

### Recipe 23
**Ingredients**

Cornu Cervi Pantotrichum, 10 g

Rhizoma Dioscoreae, 30 g

plain spirits, 500 ml

**Process**   Cut pilose antler into slices, soak them along with Chinese yams in plain spirits, seal the container and put it in a cool, dry place for seven days. Then remove the dregs (stored up for later use) and store the tincture up for future administration.

**Directions**   Take 10 ml before meals three times daily.

**Indications**   Insufficiency of both blood and essence in courses of consumptive diseases.

**Recipe** 24
**Ingredients**
Radix Stemonae, 60 g

plain spirits, 500 ml

**Process**   Cut tubers of stemona root into pieces and stir-fry them until they are done. Fill them in a gauze bag, fasten its mouth, soak it in plain spirits, seal the container and put it in a cool, dry place for seven days. Then remove the bag and store the tincture up for future administration.

**Directions**   Take 5 ml three times daily.

**Indications**   Shortness of breath, either aversion to cold or hectic fever accompanied with feverish sensation in the palms and soles.

**Recipe** 25
**Ingredients**
Cordyceps, 30 g

plain spirits, 500 ml

**Process**   Soak Chinese caterpillar fungi in plain spirits, seal the container and put it in a cool, dry place for seven days. Then remove the dregs (stored up for later use) and store the tincture up for future administration.

**Directions**   Take 10 ml twice to three times daily.

**Indication**   General weakness.

**Recipe** 26
**Ingredients**
Ganoderma Lucidum, 30 g

plain spirits, 500 ml

**Process**   Cut the first ingredient into pieces and soak them in plain spirits, seal the container and put it in a cool, dry place for fifteen days. Shake the container several times daily during soaking. Then remove the dregs (stored up for later use) and store the tincture up for future administration.

**Directions**   Take 10 ml twice daily.

**Indication**   General weakness.

**Recipe** 27
**Ingredients**
Radix Polygoni Multiflori, 60 g

plain spirits, 500 ml

**Process**   Cut the first ingredient into pieces and soak them in plain spirits, seal the container and put it in a cool, dry place for five to seven days. Shake the container several times daily during soaking. Then remove the dregs (stored up for later use) and store the tincture up for future administration.

**Directions**   Take 10 ml twice daily.

**Indication**   General weakness.

### Recipe 28
**Ingredients**

Fructus Crataegi, 250 g

Arillus Longan, 250 g

Fructus Jujubae, 30 g

brown sugar, 30 g

rice wine, 1000 ml

**Process**   Soak the first four ingredients in rice wine, seal the container and put it in a cool, dry place for five to ten days. Shake the container several times daily during soaking. Then remove the dregs (stored up for later use) and store the tincture up for future administration.

**Directions**   Take 30 ml at bedtime daily.

**Indication**   General weakness. Contraindicated for cases with constipation due to sthenic-heat retention in the intestine.

### Recipe 29
**Ingredients**

Anguilla Japonica, 1000 g

millet wine, 100 ml

**Process**   Wash the eels clean and cut them into thin pieces, put them in an earthenware pot and add in millet wine, cook the eels until they are done.

**Directions**   Take 100 g of the eels with a right amount of vinegar as a condiment, daily.

**Indication**   General weakness.

（京）新登字 207 号

**图书在版编目(CIP)数据**

中国酒疗＝CHINESE MEDICATED LIQUOR THERAPY：英文／宋农主编. - 北京：北京科学技术出版社，1996.3
ISBN 7-5304-1845-9

I. 中… II. 宋… III. 酒-食物疗法-中国-英文 IV. R247.1

中国版本图书馆 CIP 数据核字(96)第 04464 号

## 中国酒疗

主编 宋 农

翻译 李国华

北京科学技术出版社出版
（中国北京西直门南大街 16 号）
邮政编码 100035
华北矿专印刷厂印刷
中国国际图书贸易总公司发行
（中国北京车公庄西路 35 号）
北京邮政信箱第 399 号 邮政编码 100044
英文版 16 开本
1996 年 3 月第一版第一次印刷
ISBN 7-5304-1845-9/R・356

05850
14-E-2941P